Essentials of Clinical
Electric Response Audiometry

To Gemma

Essentials of Clinical Electric Response Audiometry

W.P.R. Gibson MD FRCS

Consultant ENT Surgeon,
The National Hospitals for Nervous Diseases,
London

Foreword by R.J. Ruben MD

Professor and Chairman,
Albert Einstein College of Medicine
of Yeshiva University, New York

CHURCHILL LIVINGSTONE
EDINBURGH LONDON AND NEW YORK 1978

CHURCHILL LIVINGSTONE
Medical Division of Longman Group Limited

Distributed in the United States of America by
Longman Inc., 19 West 44th Street, New York,
N.Y. 10036 and by associated companies,
branches and respresentatives throughout
the world.

First Published 1978

ISBN 0 443 01322 5

British Library Cataloguing Publication Data

Gibson, W P R
    Essentials of clinical electric response audiometry.
    1. Audiometry   2. Evoked potentials (Electrophysiology)
    I. Title
    617.8'9   RF 294   77–30317

Printed in Great Britain by
T. & A. Constable Ltd., Edinburgh

Foreword

The clinical utilisation of the electrophysiology of the auditory system has opened a new era in our ability to diagnose receptive auditory impairment. This work has been developed in the main during the last three decades by researchers in various disciplines throughout the world. The clinician now has available electrophysiological techniques with which the auditory system may be accurately and systematically evaluated. It is now possible to measure, by recording electrical potentials, the responses of the hair cells of the inner ear, the VIIIth nerve, the auditory nuclei of the brain stem, midbrain, thalamus, and the auditory cortex in most patients.

The significance of these electrophysiological measurements is manifested by our present ability to determine at what level or levels in the auditory system there is a deficit. Additionally, a statement can be made not only about where the deficit or deficits occur but also, in many instances, as to the amount of function which is present. Thus the utilisation of these electrophysiological results allows for both a qualitative and a quantitative assessment of the auditory system.

Another aspect of the application of electrophysiology to the clinical problems of the auditory system is that the large repository of data which has been accumulated in nonhuman studies has now become clinically relevant. At the present time, this archive of information is just beginning to be applied to the understanding of human receptive hearing disorders. During the next decade there should be, based on the already accumulated information, even a greater understanding of the mechanisms of the multitudinous diseases affecting the auditory system. Additionally, it is predicted that various unique and heretofore unaccountable electrophysiological responses will be observed in patients. These will form the basis for fundamental investigations in other animals. The correlation of the clinical observations and the controlled, planned animal experimentation should result both in a better understanding of the disease processes and also of the fundamental physiology of audition. It is evident that this increased understanding will lead to the efficacious intervention, care, and perhaps cure of these diseases.

It has been almost 200 years since Galvani discovered the electrical activity of biological tissue. Today we are able to apply this fundamental discovery to the entire auditory system. Every patient, infant, child or adult, no matter how impaired, can now have the auditory system objectively evaluated. Many of these patients, in the past, could not be tested by psychophysical techniques or would have to wait many years before their auditory systems could be assessed; consequently, the infant would lose the critical years for language development. Now, any and all of these patients may be evaluated and data obtained which is of a degree of accuracy upon which proper habilitative interventions can be undertaken. The advanced maturation of the electrophysiological evaluation of the auditory system can now and will continue to improve the quality of life of those individuals with receptive auditory impairments.

R. J. Ruben, M.D.

Preface

The purpose of this book is to provide a practical introduction to the subject of electric response audiometry (ERA) for otologists, audiologists and other interested groups who may wish to include ERA as part of their clinical service. An attempt has been made to review all the currently popular tests in a simple straight-forward manner beginning with basic principles. Physicists and electrical engineers will, no doubt, find that their particular fields have been incompletely mentioned as this book is written primarily for the clinician. Nevertheless it is hoped that they will find this book of interest, perhaps it will help them to understand the clinical aspects more completely. It should always be remembered that it was only due to close co-operation between scientists and clinicians that ERA emerged as a valuable tool and so anyone endeavouring to undertake these tests is well-advised to ensure that close and friendly relationships are available.

The term 'electric response audiometry' was finally accepted at the second meeting of The International ERA Study Group in Vienna (Davis, 1971). The original term 'evoked response audiometry' was thought inexact as it can reasonably be said that any test of hearing which produces a reaction from the patient, either objectively or subjectively, is a form of 'evoked response audiometry'. The use of the word 'electric' is more precise as it is the bio–electric responses from the patient which are measured in ERA.

It is much more difficult to justify the word 'audiometry' when describing ERA. Audiometry is a word formed by joining a Latin root (*audire*—to hear) to a Greek suffix (*metria*—measuring). Hearing is a psychophysical phenomenon which involves the ability not only to detect a sound but also to associate it within the brain to certain memories so that the sound becomes meaningful. The fact that a sound has evoked an electric response within the cortex of the brain does not necessarily ensure that the subject has actually heard the sound. If 'audiometry' is the measurement of hearing, then the term 'ERA' is misleading since none of the tests, with a possible exception of long latency responses such as the contingent negative variation, measures the entire process. To justify the term 'ERA' it is necessary to accept a less precise definition of 'audiometry'; namely, measurement of hearing or some part of the hearing mechanism. Whether this latter definition is acceptable or not will continue to be a source of debate but in the meantime there is no doubt that the term 'ERA' has been widely accepted.

ERA is often referred to as an 'objective test'. Audiologists commonly classify the various audiometric tests available into subjective, behavioural and objective categories. Subjective audiometry is a description of those tests which require the subject to give a voluntary response. For instance, the subject may be asked to operate a switch whenever a sound is audible. Behavioural tests monitor the reactions of the patient when influenced by sound. The young child may turn hungrily towards the noise of a spoon rattling inside a cup. These behavioural tests are partly involuntary as the child turns instinctively, and partly voluntary as the child can choose whether he is interested enough to merit the effort of turning. Objective tests require no active co-operation from the subject who can only influence the results by interfering with the test procedure. The objectivity usually only relates to the subject as often the results may require considerable 'subjective' interpretation, as does an electroencephalogram. This classification is not without its critics. Psychologists would accept any voluntary or behavioural response as a source of objective data (Bamford, 1977), whilst engineers may argue that true objectivity requires a machine capable of analysing the results without the need for any human judgement.

London 1978   W.P.R.G.

Acknowledgements

So many colleagues have helped me so much during the past three years while I have been compiling this book that it is impossible to give full mention to them all. The work was done during my appointment as senior registrar at The London Hospital and I must start by thanking the consultant staff, Andrew Morrison, John Booth and Peter McKelvie for all their encouragement during this period.

My other colleagues at The London Hospital deserve special mention. David Moffat has been an enthusiastic member of the team as has Richard Ramsden. Richard Ramsden and his wife, Wendy, have painstakingly corrected my poor grammar.

Mrs Nancy Hibbs has typed the many manuscripts. Roger Thornton and Gordon Sharrard have given me a good deal of their expert advice. John Groves, who first directed my interest towards ERA, has helped edit my literary attempts and I would like to thank him for all the help he has given me over the past years.

It has been a great privilege to work with Harry Beagley. His expert knowledge of the entire subject has been invaluable and I cannot thank him enough for all the help he has given me both with my own research projects and with the writing of this book. We have had the opportunity of working together for several years and he has always been a very kind and understanding co-worker.

Lastly, I must mention my wife and children who have provided the atmosphere of love which has kept me going during the many hours of writing. Without their help this book would have been impossible.

W.P.R.G.

Contents

Introduction

The clinical uses of ERA

There are three main applications for ERA within the clinic:

1. As a means of estimating hearing acuity.
2. As a method of diagnosis—identifying the cause of a hearing defect or detecting some lesion which is affecting the auditory pathway.
3. As a means of monitoring the effects of surgical or pharmacological intervention upon the auditory mechanism.

1. As a measure of hearing acuity. There are several methods of ERA which provide a means of assessing the function of certain levels of the auditory system and these tests can be used to estimate the hearing acuity. There are two groups of patients in which an objective test of auditory function is especially helpful.

The first and most obvious group is young children. The need for an objective test is particularly evident in small children with multiple handicaps such as cerebral palsy and blindness, as these children can prove difficult to assess with certainty using conventional behavioural techniques. It can be hoped that when two methods of assessment are used, behavioural and objective, less serious errors will result. When the two methods are not in complete agreement, the need for further careful testing is readily apparent. It is most unwise to place entire reliance on objective tests in the face of conflicting clinical evidence. It is always possible that the machine was faulty or that it was recording an artefact which was mistaken for a true response. It is sensible only to use objective audiometric tests as part of a battery of investigations. The availability of such tests should not be allowed to lead to any erosion of standards of clinical testing but should enhance the expertise of the workers involved.

The second group is adults. These subjects may be divided into two categories: firstly, subjects with dementia or other handicaps which make it difficult for them to give subjective responses; secondly, subjects with non-organic hearing problems. When a clinical diagnosis of a non-organic hearing loss is reached, it is very helpful to have available some objective test which can check the diagnosis. With the welcome arrival in Britain, as in other parts of the world, of legislation for compensation of industrial noise induced hearing loss, the need for a simple objective test has become more vital.

2. As a method of diagnosis. Audiometric tests not only provide a measure of hearing acuity but also give important information which can be used to learn more about the nature of the hearing defect. ERA is no exception and, indeed, it may even give valuable information about physiological activity outside the auditory system.

1

Most of the responses used for ERA show the function of a particular part of the auditory pathway. The electrocochleogram tells much about the activity of the cochlea and eighth nerve. Brainstem electrical responses reveal the passage of electrical stimulation through important areas of the brainstem and are rapidly becoming a useful neurological tool. Similarly, the other methods of ERA mentioned in this book show the function of various parts of the auditory mechanism. It is often helpful to combine the results from several different tests as such a combination may reveal more accurately the exact site of auditory dysfunction.

3. As a means of monitoring the effects of surgery or pharmacological agents. In animal work, the electrical responses derived from various parts of the auditory system have been used for several years to monitor the effect of surgery or drugs. In human work, this field is comparatively unexplored. It does seem likely that tests such as electrocochleography will provide a means of assessing the effect of various treatments on the patients themselves. This avenue of investigation may prove particularly helpful in the understanding of pathological conditions, such as Ménière's disorder and forms of tinnitus, for which there is no true animal model.

Finally, there seems little doubt that ERA can offer a great deal to the clinician. The technical advances within the past 20 years have been dramatic and it is hoped that over the next few years, the clinical aspects of ERA will advance accordingly.

1. The History and Development of ERA

The presence of electrical potentials in the brain was first noted by Caton (1875) who managed to record electrical changes in the exposed brain of rabbits and monkeys. Despite extensive investigation of the functions of the nervous system, it was not until over fifty years later that Hans Berger, a neurologist from Jena, recorded the first human electroencephalogram (EEG) from electrodes placed on the scalp (Berger, 1929). There was initial reluctance by physiologists to accept Berger's findings as they doubted the reliability of his technique. He had used a simple galvanometer which was not able to measure accurately voltages as minute as those obtained from the surface of the scalp and an optical recording system which was itself prone to error.

Berger (1930) described a change in the rhythm of the electroencephalogram when he either dropped a steel ball into a dish or exploded a fire cracker to produce a sudden loud noise. He was fascinated more, however, by the first electrical rhythm that he had described which is now known as *alpha* rhythm. He noted that at rest the electroencephalogram was characterised by large slightly irregular waves occurring at the rate of 8-12 per second. If the subject opened his eyes or began some mental activity, then this rhythm was inhibited and smaller, faster waves replaced it. It worried physiologists at the time that the largest brain activity should be recorded whilst the brain was resting. It was felt therefore by many that Berger's recordings were artefacts and it was only after the work of Adrian and Matthews (1934) that their scepticism was refuted. Adrian and Matthews (1934) used a valve amplifier and an accurate pen recording apparatus which left no doubt as to the authenticity of Berger's work. Adrian himself suggested that the *alpha* rhythm should be known also as the *Berger* rhythm in respect for the discoverer.

Electroencephalographic audiometry

Following Berger's earlier work, several workers attempted to identify specific changes in the electroencephalogram in response to tactile, visual or auditory stimulation but their work was hampered since the specific changes were largely obscured by the background fluctuations of the other EEG waves. Loomis, Harvey and Hobart (1938) described diphasic or triphasic potentials which occurred at the vertex of the head in response to tactile stimulation during sleep. In the next year, P.A. Davis (1939) and H. Davis and his co-workers (1939) reported similar responses to auditory stimuli. The advent of the second world war prevented further research but once the war had ended several groups of workers became involved in the field.

It appears that there are at least four different effects that indicate that the EEG is being altered by auditory stimulation (Derbyshire and McDermott, 1958). Firstly there is an *on* response which is larger in sleep, related to the switching on of the sound stimulus, with a latency between 50-500 ms. This was the response first described by P.A. Davis (1939). Later the response became known as the *vertex potential* or *V potential* and it is the response electronically averaged in CERA. Secondly, there is a reduction in voltage of, particularly, the faster frequencies of the EEG with a latency of 200-600 ms. Thirdly, there are frequent *off* effects which may be larger than the *on* effects when very quiet sounds are used. The *off* effects consist of brief periods of voltage reduction related to the switching off of the sound stimulus. Finally, there is the *late* effect occurring about 25 seconds after a pure tone burst of about 4 seconds' duration. This is a relatively sudden change in the entire pattern of the electroencephalogram signifying an alteration in the level of consciousness.

Many difficulties were unfortunately encountered when attempts were made to use these findings as the basis of a clinical test. To produce results with any reliability it was necessary, especially in children, to test the subjects whilst drowsy from either natural or induced sleep. In addition to the clinical difficulties of monitoring the level of consciousness and the long time it took to obtain the recordings, the results required prolonged analysis after the session to decide which changes had been due to the auditory stimuli and which changes were due to unrelated events. In view of all these problems it is hardly surprising that the method never gained much clinical acceptance.

Psychogalvanic (electrodermal) skin resistance audiometry

In the immediate post-war period whilst some workers were developing electroencephalographic audiometry, others, notably Bordley and Hardy of the Hearing and Speech Center at Baltimore (Bordley and Hardy, 1949: Bordley, Hardy and Richter, 1948), were responsible for applying the phenomena of skin resistance changes to audiometry and for evolving a practical procedure for testing the hearing of young children. Psychogalvanic skin resistance (PGSR) audiometry is also known by the term *electrodermal audiometry (EDA)*. The advantages of this method were that the apparatus involved was relatively simple and the results often clear-cut. Initially PGSR audiometry was the most promising technique available (Doerfler, 1948).

There are two basic methods of assessing the psychogalvanic reflex (Lindsley, 1963). The endosomatic method was suggested by Tarchanoff (1890) and measures the difference in electrical potential arising from currents in the skin. The currents are of extremely low magnitude and require DC amplifiers of high sensitivity and stability. Since these amplifiers were not available in the early 1950's, little work was done using this method. The second method, named the exosomatic method, uses the method suggested by Vigoroux (1879) and later by Feré (1888). This involves the application of electric current with a low voltage potential between the electrodes and measuring the change of resistance directly from the electrodes. This change in skin resistance only occurs with very loud sounds and is therefore of limited value in the determination of auditory thresholds. If, however, the subject is *conditioned* to the stimulus, then responses may be obtained using near threshold sounds and the test becomes much more useful clinically. The change in skin resistance is due to an increase in the activity of sudoriferous (sweat) glands in response to increased activity of the sympathetic nervous system. The secretion or sweat produced conducts electricity well, so that the resistance between the two electrodes on the skin surface is diminished. To enhance this activity, use is made of a type of Pavlovian conditioned reflex. It will be recalled that Pavlov's experiment (Pavlov, 1927) involved dogs which salivated (*unconditioned response*) at the sight of their food (*unconditioned stimulus*). Pavlov sounded a bell (*conditioned stimulus*) immediately before the dogs were given their food and after several of these *conditioning* meal-times, the poor dogs salivated whenever the bell was sounded even though their food was not presented. In PGSR audiometry, the sweating (*unconditioned response*) is stimulated by an electric shock (*unconditioned stimulus*) and the *conditioned stimulus* is a pure tone signal. After the subject has received several electric shocks which are unpleasant enough to make him sweat and that are associated with a pure tone, it is found that he becomes conditioned and sweats in response to the sound alone.

Originally it was hoped that the sweating response was analogous to the finger raising response in adults. In other words, instead of the child having to move a toy or raise his hand, a positive PGSR response meant that the signal had been heard. Bordley (1956), however, believed that the auditory-sympathetic reflex involved did not involve the auditory cortex and that a positive PGSR response did not necessarily mean that the sound was being perceived. In 1954, Wang had established the level of the shock-sweat reflex in cats by transecting the animal's brain at different levels. He found that transection at intercollicular level to the rostral border of the pons abolished the reflex, whilst transection above this level left the reflex intact. The auditory-sympathetic reflex must lie somewhere between the cortex and the level of the inferior colliculi. It is therefore evident that PGSR can only demonstrate that the auditory pathway is intact up to this level and does not show that the sound has reached the cortex or is being understood.

PGSR audiometry was harmed by some of the initially over-enthusiastic reports which appeared in the literature. It was soon discovered that PGSR was not the panacea which some workers expected and as a result the pendulum of opinion swung against the test and some highly critical reports were written. For instance, it was discovered that the procedure was of the least value in the cases in which it was most needed. The same group of children that were difficult to test by conventional behavioural means proved to be the most difficult to test using PGSR.

During the test period it is necessary to keep extraneous physical movements to a minimum since such activity results in changes of skin resistance which are difficult to differentiate from the true PGSR responses to the sound stimuli. Children with brain damage and severe neurological defects are often troubled by jerky or vermicular involuntary movements which make the procedure impractical. Many other young children, especially those that suffer psychological difficulties, find the procedure too lengthy and cannot maintain their cooperation. These children struggle and disturb the electrodes or burst into tears. Sometimes children are upset by the conditioning shocks and the test has to be concluded before it has even begun.

Often in children, it is difficult to determine whether or not the conditioning has been carried out correctly. If a child is really severely deaf, all that may be achieved is that he receives a series of unpleasant electric shocks without ever hearing the pure tones with which they are to be associated. Even when correct conditioning has been obtained, habituation may occur. The subject, realising that no more shocks are being given with the sounds, stops sweating. Barr (1955) gives a detailed description of the technique involved and of the difficulties encountered on testing children. He concluded that the method was extremely time-consuming, and was based, 'for the children as well as the examiners', on an unpleasant experience.

Now that the true value of PGSR audiometry has been realised, it is possible that it may be accepted again for the evaluation of certain specific clinical problems. The advantage of PGSR is that the equipment needed is relatively cheap and simple and can be used by non-medical personnel. The results are usually clear-cut although when testing adults a constant watch for habituation has to be kept. The most relevant application of PGSR is probably in the detection of non-organic or functional hearing losses. If the new laws based on the report by the Industrial Injuries Advisory Council (1973) result in an increase of such cases, then it is likely that audiologists will be forced to employ objective means of verifying the results obtained by pure tone audiometry. At present, only CERA and PGSR employ pure tones as the stimulus and give results which can be compared directly with the pure tone audiogram.

Psychogalvanic skin resistance audiometry is not discussed further in this book in view of its present limited clinical usage. Any reader wishing to learn more about the matter is advised to read the authoritative accounts by Knox (1972) and Ventry (1975).

The introduction of averaging techniques

It was the introduction of electronic averaging techniques that entirely revolutionised the science of electric response audiometry (ERA). Until such techniques were available, the main problem of using the electroencephalogram remained that of detecting the response to a stimulus when the background noise was of greater amplitude than that of the specific electrical event. Methods involving the superimposition of EEG tracings, either ink written or using photographs (Dawson, 1947, 1950; Abé, 1954), did not in practice allow more than 10–20 responses to be used.

Electronic averaging allows the investigator to accumulate as many responses as he wishes. The essential points are described in Chapter 2. The bioelectric response evoked by a particular stimulus always occurs after the same time interval. If the electrical events are recorded on an oscilloscope, the evoked electric response will occur at a specific point of the sweep on each occasion. When a single response is obtained, it is difficult to detect it because of the background fluctuations. If, however, the separate sweeps to successive identical stimuli are added together, then the response being time-locked grows larger whilst the background fluctuations, being random in nature, gradually cancel themselves out. It was Dr J.N. Hunt who first suggested this additive technique and his co-worker at The National Hospitals for Nervous Diseases, Dr G.D. Dawson (1951, 1954) who brilliantly exploited it. Dawson used the method to detect visual and tactile stimuli. Unhappily, no work in England was done with acoustic stimuli using this method.

Some years later, Clark (1958) and his co-workers (Clark et al., 1962) developed an 'average response computer'. This device converts analog data into a digital form from which averages, amplitudes and time histograms can easily be computed. This form of 'digital averaging' is favoured by most ERA workers today.

The myogenic 'sonomotor' responses (Chapter 6)

When Geisler, Frishkopf and Rosenblith (1958) first applied electronic averaging to the detection of auditory evoked responses, they placed their electrodes on the surface of the scalp. They discovered responses with short latencies (the time between the stimulus and the response) of 8–30 ms (milliseconds). Geisler, on the basis of his own animal experiments on monkeys (Geisler, 1960) and those of other workers (Jarcho, 1949; Chang, 1950; inter alia) believed that these responses were most probably derived from the primary auditory cortex. He noted that they could be obtained from electrode sites all over the scalp but surprisingly the largest potentials were found at the inion, which is the small, bony protuberance at the back of the skull. The amplitude or size of the potentials varied widely even in the same subject, especially on adopting different head positions, and so he took steps to exclude the possibility of myogenic contamination. Later, he even used a piezo-electric crystal device which was sensitive to shifts of as little as 5×10^{-6} mm (Geisler, 1964), but he was unable to detect any movement of the scalp musculature to even the loudest of sounds.

In 1963, Bickford and his colleagues (Bickford, Galbraith and Jacobson, 1963a; Bickford, Jacobson and Galbraith, 1963b) published their work which showed without much doubt that the source of the response was muscle. Using clicks of 100–135 dB SL, they detected responses not only from the scalp muscles but also from the facial and limb musculature. They (Bickford, Jacobson and Cody, 1964) distinguished the inion response (latency 8–10 ms) from the startle response to a pistol shot (latency 25 ms) and the voluntary response (latency 100 ms). They proposed the presence of an audiomotor (sonomotor) system and coined the term audiomyoclonus as an analogy to photomyoclonus which had previously been described by Bickford et al. (1952). They showed (Bickford et al., 1964; Cody et al., 1964) that administration of curare could, with the notable exception of the parietal response, completely abolish the responses. Furthermore, in three deaf patients with normal vestibular function, they managed to record responses from the inion. Later, when the cortical responses to auditory stimuli had been discovered, it was suggested (Davis *et al*., 1963) that responses occurring within 50 ms of the stimulus should be known as fast, to distinguish them from the slow responses which occurred after this time.

Once the truly cortical responses had been identified, it was not surprising that workers turned to this more promising field. The myogenic responses are indirect as they involve structures that are not necessary to hearing and they are limited in only demonstrating that the lower auditory pathways are intact. Worse still, the work of Cody and Bickford (Cody *et al*., 1964) had shown that responses might be obtained by stimulating the vestibular receptors alone so that a clinician would be led to believe that a patient was hearing when in fact he was totally deaf. Despite the apparent unattractiveness of the myogenic responses, no biological phenomenon should be totally ignored and further interest in the myogenic responses has been raised sporadically. In particular, it is the muscle responses which can be obtained from the inion, parietal area and the post-auricular area that have proved the most fascinating.

The Inion Response

All attempts to use this response to indicate auditory thresholds were abandoned once it had been shown that stimulation of vestibular receptors could evoke it. Cody and Bickford (1969) have demonstrated that the inion response may be evoked, albeit at different latencies, by visual and tactile stimuli as well as by sounds. Davis (1965a) believed that when sound was employed at moderate intensities only the cochlear pathway was involved. Ruhm and Flanigin (1967) suggested the presence of a cochleo-neurogenic response at low intensities and a vestibulo-myogenic response at high intensities but there is no evidence to suggest that this response is anything but myogenic, and later evidence suggests that the neural element was being recorded from the reference vertex electrode.

Attempts have been made to use the inion response as an objective method of assessing vestibular function (Tabor, Best and Metz, 1968; Pignatro, 1972) but the results have not been promising. The author (Gibson, 1974) found that the presence or size of the inion response correlated poorly with the results obtained by caloric testing. He believed that the most likely explanation was that when the vestibular system was involved, it was unlikely that the response originated from the cristae of the lateral semi-circular canal and more probable that it involved the otolith organ (either the saccule or utricle).

The Parietal Response

Goldstein and Rodman (1967) used this response for objective audiometry. They claimed that they could detect responses to within 5 dB of the subjective auditory threshold in 55 per cent of a group of 20 normal subjects. Other workers have supported the concept of a neurogenic origin of an early response and found it to be centred at the vertex (Borsanyi and Blanchard, 1964; Lowell, 1965; Ruhm and Flanigin, 1967). It is this potential that currently is being expertly exploited by Mendel and Hosick (1975) amongst others (Chapter Eight).

The Post-Auricular Response

Kiang and co-workers (1963) first reported the post-auricular myogenic response which has a peak latency of approximately 15 ms. They managed to obtain results using clicks of low intensity in 80 per cent of a group of normally hearing subjects, and could not obtain the response in two patients that were deaf. The response could be obtained even using clicks occurring at a rate of 200 per second. However, they found the response exasperating as subjects appeared to grow accustomed to the test procedure and then stopped giving responses. They managed to recover the response by giving their subjects electric shocks to their feet! Although Jacobson et al., (1964) stated that the response showed no sign of fatigue, both Kiang et al., (1963) and Davis et al., (1963) have illustrated their texts with examples which showed rapid habituation. Gibson (1974) found that the response did not fatigue in a uniform manner but that it diminished as the subject relaxed and enlarged when the subject was alerted.

The post-auricular response is extremely variable and can be difficult to obtain in some subjects. Cody and Bickford (1969) used tone bursts (with a rise time of 1 ms) presented twice each second and tested 60 normal volunteers. In four of these subjects, they were unable to obtain the response from either ear even on using clicks with intensities of 110 dB SL and in the remaining 112 ears tested, a further 15 did not yield a response. On average, a tone burst of 90 dB was necessary before the response could be identified. On the basis of this study, they concluded that measurement of the post-auricular response could not be used as a method of assessing auditory acuity. Yoshie and Okudaira (1969), however, used clicks and found the response to be consistent and managed to identify responses in the majority of their subjects quite close to the auditory thresholds. They concluded that the post-auricular response could be used not only as an indicator for objective audiometry but also as a means of demonstrating the integrity of the neural pathways concerned within the brainstem. Milner (1970) in her study of the cortical auditory responses reported in detail how she found that the post-auricular response provided a useful check on the results she had obtained.

Gibson (1974) evaluated the basic properties of this response and found the most likely explanation for the differing conclusions reached by various workers lay with the type of stimulus they employed. It appears that the response can only be evoked consistently by clicks with a very abrupt onset. Douek, Gibson and Humphries (1973) found that the largest potentials were obtained if the active electrode was placed in the middle of the post-auricular muscle and the reference electrode on the edge of it. The response had to be obtained bilaterally and simultaneously, as it was quite unpredictable which side would yield the clearer potential. To emphasise the existence of a contralateral response as well as an ipsilateral response, they named the post-auricular myogenic response when obtained, with the electrode positions specified, from both sides simultaneously the crossed acoustic response. Although most clinicians like the term on account of its simplicity, audiologists experienced in the field of objective audiometry have rightly pointed out that it may mislead a reader into believing that the response may only be obtained from the contralateral side to the ear being stimulated.

Douek et al., (1973) managed to detect abnormalities of the response in patients with brainstem lesions and have suggested that it may have a use in detecting such lesions. By incorporating a device which excluded any gross movement artefacts from the recordings, they (Douek, Gibson and Humphries, 1974) managed to obtain potentials from even unco-operative young children without sedation and this allowed a prediction of the hearing acuity actually to be made during clinics. More recently, Ashcroft, Humphries and Douek (1975) have used the *crossed acoustic test* objectively to assess the hearing status of neonates.

Cortical electric response audiometry (CERA) (Chapter 3)

During the period between 1963 and 1972, the vast majority of workers were concerned with the measurement of the slow evoked auditory response which has been shown to be definitely cortical in nature. It had been P.A. Davis (1939) who first identified a triphasic or biphasic auditory evoked response in EEG recordings. Bancaud, Bloch and Paillard (1953) and Gastaut (1953) both suggested the name *V potential* to emphasise the anatomical distribution of this response which is centred around the vertex of the head.

Williams and Graham (1963) were the first to report using an electronic technique to average the *V potential* in their study performed on 21 teenagers. Nevertheless, it was Davis and Yoshie (1963), a few months later, who published the first clear account of the shape and the latency of the response, and it is surely Hallowell Davis who has taken the primary role in establishing clinically this useful method of objective audiology.

The V potential has a long duration of about 250 milliseconds in adults and it is even longer in children. It is best evoked using pure tone bursts of about 30 ms presented at 1–2 second intervals. A train of 30–60 pulses is most commonly employed and the sum of these responses is displayed in an averaged form. To discover threshold it is necessary to commence testing well above the expected level and to reduce the intensity of stimulation from trial to trial until the threshold is crossed as is shown by a clearly negative response. At levels close to threshold, the response may be difficult to identify and trials may have to be repeated to check for the consistency which indicates a truly positive response. Many factors, such as habituation, limit the normal useful test session length to about 1½ hours and so it is usual to restrict the threshold estimations to a limited number of ear-frequency combinations.

CERA in Objective Audiometry

The main advantages of CERA are that the stimulus is a pure tone so that results are directly comparable with those obtained using subjective pure tone audiometry, and the electrodes are merely fixed to the surface of the scalp without discomfort, without raising any ethical problems. Although there is a wide variation in the size of the responses obtained from different individuals, it is possible, given only the passive co-operation of the subject, to determine within a few decibels the subjective hearing thresholds (Davis *et al.*, 1967); Beagley and Kellogg, 1968; Economopoulou, Krogh and Fosvig, 1970; *inter alia*).

The main difficulties are encountered on using the response clinically in young children under seven years of age. Usually these children have been referred simply because behavioural assessment has yielded no reliable result. Even in the children who co-operate passively (Beagley, 1971 and 1972), there is usually a 20 dB gap between the objective and subjective thresholds and this gap is even greater in neonates. The amplitudes and latencies of the response in young children are most variable and this often leads to difficulties in identification (Davis et al., 1967; Cody and Townsend, 1973). Kawamura et al., (1972) advise that the averaged response should be displayed after 50, 100, 150 and 200 trials and only if it grows consistently can it be accepted as a *true* response. If a child hears only with one ear, the responses to binaural stimulation are smaller than normal.

Unfortunately, as a lot of the young children referred for this test have behavioural problems, they do not remain still for long periods without considerable coaxing. Most of the audiologists who use the test regularly possess much skill in the matter and manage to persuade the children to co-operate for a useful amount of time, but this skill only comes with experience and a casual tester may often be forced to abandon the procedure. Movements result in artefacts which may produce *false positive* results in that the artefact is mistaken for a hearing response. Such events can lead the clinician to believe that the child hears, and cause disastrous mismanagement.

In some children, a type of EEG background is encountered with large low frequency components and the technique of extracting the response by averaging may not be entirely successful. This is due to the similarity between the frequency spectrum of the background and the response itself which makes averaging less effective. This problem is worse in various forms of brain damage. It is suggested that contraindications to using CERA in young children include brain damage, muscle tics or spasms (e.g. athetosis) and epilepsy (Beagley and Gibson, 1974).

Sedation has been tried to avoid these problems but the effects of this on the response remain uncertain. A recent symposium on the subject was held in Vienna in 1971 and has been summarised by Davis (1973). One point of agreement amongst the speakers was that CERA under sedation yields responses which are more difficult and less reliable than in the waking state. However, Osterhammel, Terkildsen and Arndal (1970) found the responses clearer in deep sleep whilst Salomon et al., (1973) described deep sleep as undesirable, stating that false positives and misses (when the response is not detected) occurred too frequently to allow accurate interpretation. Obviously there is a great deal of disagreement, even amongst the experts, as to the best level and method of sedation.

All these reasons taken together probably account for the fact that, although so much has been written describing CERA, there are very few papers advocating it as a method of objective audiometry in young children.

CERA in Neuro-Otological Diagnosis

Apart from as a measurement of auditory threshold, CERA has been investigated to discover whether or not the responses may be of any value in revealing the cause or level of hearing dysfunction. Unfortunately, findings have, to date, been rather disappointing.

Davis (1972) stated that the V potential is of a secondary diffuse nature. Earlier he (Davis, 1965b) had described it as arising from the cortex over a wide area like a cap worn well forward on the head. The recordings taken directly from the surgically exposed human cortex (Sem Jacobson et al., 1956; Chatrian, Petersen and Lazarte, 1960; Celesia et al., 1968) and the recordings obtained from animals (Teas and Kiang, 1964; David and Sohmer, 1972) would appear to confirm its nature as a secondary response. Some disagreement exists (Vaughan, 1969). If one accepts that this is a secondary response, then it is not surprising that its nature is so variable and it is this variability that makes its use in neuro-otological diagnosis so uncertain.

Although CERA alone may not yet have been analysed sufficiently to be useful, it certainly can help reveal central forms of hearing dysfunction when used together with the earlier methods of ERA such as electrocochleography. Morrison, Gibson and Beagley (1976) describe a young man with a medially placed acoustic neuroma in whom the eighth nerve action potentials were normal despite the absence of subjective hearing. CERA gave no response and so it was certain that this was not a case of non-organic hearing loss but due to disruption of the auditory pathway. At present this is probably the best indication for the use of CERA in neuro-otology but it is hoped that eventually with the development of computerised data processing it will become possible to use CERA in many other ways. For instance, Arlinger (1976b) has shown differences in the latencies in 6 subjects with retrocochlear lesions using stimuli consisting of frequency ramps with different rates of frequency change.

Electrocochleography (ECochG) (Chapter 4)

At present the most acceptable abbreviation for *electrocochleography* is *ECochG* since *ECOG* has already been ascribed to the *electrocorticogram* or the measurement of cortical potentials by placing the electrodes on the exposed brain cortex.

Perhaps it is because of the difficulties encountered in the use of CERA as a clinical tool that there has been such widespread interest in the development of electrocochleography. Electrocochleography involves recording the electrical activity of the cochlear and first order, eighth nerve fibres. Adrian (1926) first recorded the action potentials of sensory nerves in animals, and later Wever and Bray (1930) managed to obtain potentials from the eighth nerve. Initially, they believed that the potentials represented a series of nerve action potentials but two years later, Saul and Davis (1932) managed to separate the true action potentials and it was discovered that these earlier recordings were of the cochlear microphonic.

The first attempts to record human cochlear potentials met with little success (Fromm, Nylen and Zotterman, 1935; Andreev, Arapora and Gerusuni, 1939; Perlman and Case, 1941) because of the minute voltages involved. Despite a promising preliminary report, Lempert Wever and Lawrence (1947) were forced to conclude that at that time the recording of cochlear potentials was not a clinical possibility (Lempert *et al.*, 1950). These workers showed great ingenuity. They were successful in most cases when they could actually place the electrode on to the round window membrane. Together with Von Békésy, they devised a special instrument made like a miniature cystoscope to enable them to place the electrode accurately through the tympanic membrane. It was, however, the anatomy of the round window hidden within its niche and directed medially that caused their main difficulties; but this problem is the very factor which makes transtympanic electrocochleography such a safe procedure today.

Technology advanced and soon Ruben *et al.*, (1960, 1961, 1963) had managed to obtain good recordings during middle ear surgery in a number of pathological conditions. Once again it was the advent of electronic averaging techniques which revolutionised the subject. Ronis (1966) was the first to use such a method during surgery but at about this time objections were raised to the test in America on ethical grounds and prevented further development in that country. In 1967, several groups of workers from all over the world described techniques for obtaining the electrocochleogram in patients not undergoing surgery. In Japan, Yoshie, Ohashi and Suzuki (1967) recorded responses from an electrode embedded in the external acoustic meatus. This method, with a slight modification, was used also by Elberling and Salomon (1971), Coats and Dickey (1970) and Khechinashvili and Kevanishvili (1974). In France, Portmann with his group (1967, 1968) obtained their potentials from a thin needle electrode which pierced the tympanic membrane to lie on the bony promontory. Sohmer and Feinmesser (1967), in Israel, used earlobe and mastoid positions for the active electrode. In Germany, Spreng and Keidel (1967) recorded from the mastoid and scalp. Later in the U.S.A., Martin and Coats (1973) recorded responses from the nasopharynx.

The cochlear potentials conduct freely through the inner ear fluids to the round window but the current is rapidly diminished by the electrically resistant tissues such as skin and bone. It is not surprising that the transtympanic electrode as used by the Portmann group yields the clearest potentials. The potentials obtained from the promontory are about 15 times larger than those from the tympanic membrane and about 50 times larger than those from the mastoid area or earlobe.

Transtympanic Electrocochleography

This method has gained widespread clinical acceptance since the responses are most distinct and there is rarely any difficulty of interpretation. It is possible to identify responses to even low levels of stimulation and this allows the auditory threshold to be estimated with a very acceptable degree of accuracy. No masking of the non-test ear is required since it is not possible to obtain the potentials from the opposite ear using such an electrode placement. Finally, the responses are unaffected by general anaesthetic agents. These properties combine to form a robust test of peripheral auditory function which may be applied to any subject possessing normal external and middle ear anatomy. Transtympanic electrocochleography offers the opportunity to determine the hearing status of subjects such as disturbed and multiple-handicapped children who, prior to the advent of this method, were impossible to test (Beagley, Hutton and Hayes, 1974).

The action potential (AP) may be obtained either using clicks or brief pure tone bursts. Due to the slow velocity of the travelling wave, the damping effect of the basilar membrane and the phase of the stimulus, low frequency tone bursts only evoke a small, poorly synchronised AP. This limits the threshold information in many subjects to frequencies of 1 kHz or higher. Some subjects do yield threshold responses at 500 Hz. This matter is discussed fully in Chapter Four.

In some countries, such as the United States of America, there are fears that the procedure of actually piercing the tympanic membrane may lead to complications and possibly expensive litigation. Crowley, Davis and Beagley (1975) published the incidence of mishaps which have occurred on using the procedure in several thousand patients at different centres throughout the world. They have shown it to be extremely safe. Interestingly, the incidence of otitis media following testing was no greater than that to be expected in a control series not tested. The author has used transtympanic electrocochleography in over four hundred adult patients and has not yet encountered any serious problems. In fact, most of the patients tested preferred the procedure to caloric testing. Since notable authorities, such as Hallowell Davis, believe the technique to be relatively harmless, no competent clinician should now fear litigation. Nevertheless, it is probably wiser to exclude patients suffering from psychiatric conditions.

Transtympanic ECochG in neuro-otological diagnosis

Electrocochleography offers far more than the mere estimation of the auditory threshold. It offers a unique picture of the electrical function of the ear in health and disease. Using a transtympanic electrode, three different types of electrical response may be recorded. These are the compound nerve action potential which is used for judging the auditory threshold, and the summating potential (SP) and the cochlear microphonics (CM) which are not directly related to hearing acuity.

The action potential when obtained from the same ear is a reliable and exact indicator of cochlear function. The size (amplitude) and timing (latency) of the response alter with changes in the intensity of the stimulation. These changes may be plotted as input/output graphs which reveal important differences between conductive, recruiting and other hearing pathologies (Charlet de Sauvage and Aran, 1973). The shape of the response is also consistent. The normal response is monophasic and this form is also encountered in cases of conductive deafness, but in some cases of sensory or cochlear deafness, the response becomes diphasic. In most cases of neural deafness, the potential is prolonged by the superimposition of a slow DC component and, interestingly, an enhanced SP results in a similar waveform in patients with Ménière's disorder (Gibson and Beagley, 1976b). These patterns and others will be described in more detail in Chapter Four.

Electrocochleography from the surface of the tympanic membrane

It is possible to obtain potentials from the surface of the tympanic membrane without piercing it. Cullen et al., (1972) twisted a pledglet of cotton wool soaked in saline on to the end of an electrode and placed this on the surface of the ear drum. Similarly, Humphries, Ashcroft and Douek (1977) have used a silver ball electrode. Unfortunately, the action potential is much smaller when averaged from this site. Sohmer and Feinmesser (1964) found that the action potential in the cat was approximately 10 times smaller when obtained from the tympanic membrane rather than from the round window. On account of the size of the potentials, most workers have had difficulty in tracing them using stimuli of less than 50 dB above the auditory threshold. Placing an electrode on the surface of the tympanic membrane requires more surgical skill than simply piercing it. Obviously, this method is unsuitable for young children without using sedation, and if the child has to undergo an anaesthetic it is reasonable to use a trans-tympanic electrode position to achieve the best possible conditions for obtaining a significant result (Berlin *et al.*, 1974).

Electrocochleography from the external acoustic meatus
Although Yoshie *et al.* (1967) originally placed their active electrode under the surface of the posterior wall of the external acoustic meatus, they now favour the transtympanic method. Coats and Dickey (1970) placed a needle electrode into the meatus close to the annulus and recorded both action potentials and cochlear microphonics. They were able to demonstrate many of the functions of the response and compare them to recordings obtained in cats. However, piercing the meatal wall is as painful as piercing the tympanic membrane. Montandon *et al.* (1975a, b) have developed a technique for obtaining the recordings from the surface of the meatus using a silver foil disc. These workers were able to obtain responses at 40 dB peak SPL in a group of normal subjects and believe that this technique can be used as a clinic procedure.

Electrocochleography from other external sites
The action potential from the first order cochlear nerve fibres and the cochlear microphonics may be recorded from distant sites which include: the hard palate (Keidel, 1971b), the ear lobe (Sohmer and Feinmesser, 1970) and the mastoid (Jewett and Williston, 1971; Hecox and Galambos, 1974). These recordings, however, offer far more than measurement of cochlear function as it is possible to obtain a series of waves with longer latencies which arise from important auditory areas within the brainstem. Hecox and Galambos (1974) used the term *brainstem auditory evoked responses* which is a much better description than electrocochleography, as this misleads one to believe that only the electrical output of the cochlea is being measured.

The auditory brainstem electrical responses (ber)
(Chapter 5)

Most workers obtain these responses by placing the active electrode either on the mastoid skin or on the earlobe and positioning the reference electrode on the surface of the scalp at the vertex or the midline of the forehead immediately beneath the hairline. There is a series of five or more deflections that may be recorded from these sites (Jewett, Romano and Williston, 1970; Sohmer and Feinmesser, 1971; Thornton, 1975a). Lev and Sohmer (1972) compared the experimental results obtained in cats with human recordings and postulated the relation of each wave to important parts of the auditory tract. The first wave seems to be identical with the response in transtympanic electrocochleography and is the action potential of the first order cochlear nerve fibres. The second wave is generated in the cochlear nucleus, the third in the superior olivary complex and the fourth and fifth in the inferior colliculus. Buchwald and Huang (1975) more recently related the fourth wave to the ventral nucleus of lateral lemniscus and pre-olivary region.

The auditory brainstem responses have been used as a method of threshold audiometry (Sohmer and Feinmesser, 1973; Terkildsen, Osterhammel and Huis in't Veld, 1973). The first wave is usually very small, being less than a millionth of a volt, and may be very difficult to trace using low intensities of acoustic stimulation. The fifth wave (Jewett classification [Jewett *et al.*, 1970]), nevertheless, is an excellent measure of auditory acuity which may be traced to levels of 5–15 dB SL.

The most valuable application of these responses will lie, perhaps, in the neuro-otological field. Sohmer, Feinmesser and Szabo (1974) have found that, in cases with known brainstem lesions, it is possible to determine the point at which the auditory tract is damaged by noting the number of waves which remain intact. For instance, in the case of a patient with a petrous bone meningioma, only the first two deflections were visible. Starr and Achor (1975) have published similar findings in a large number of patients with various central lesions. Further details are given in Chapter 5.

The Cochlear microphonics (CM) and summating potential (SP)

Apart from the action potentials arising from the eighth nerve, two of the other electrical phenomena resulting from sound stimulation within the normal cochlea can be recorded. These are the cochlear microphonics (CM) and summating potential (SP). The CM have waveforms which closely resemble the electrical waveform of the acoustic stimulus—the CM evoked by a 500 Hz stimulus are difficult to distinguish from the shape of the stimulus itself. The CM recorded from the promontory closely follow the movements of the basilar membrane (Dallos, 1972) and can be attributed, therefore, mainly to the displacement-sensitive outer hair cells.

It is a problem that the cochlear microphonics should reproduce so faithfully the waveform of the stimulus, as it is difficult to separate the 'true CM' from 'pseudo-CM' caused by the induction phenomena of an alternating current flow in the acoustic stimulating system (Yoshie and Yamaura, 1969). The other property of CM that makes their use in audiometry less certain is that they have no threshold. If CM are present, then it is possible to produce a recording using any intensity of stimulation providing the apparatus is sensitive enough.

The CM recorded from the promontory relate only to the hair cells lying closest to the round window membrane. The chief reason is the phase characteristics of CM; the hair cells along the cochlear partition produce CM in different phases so that the net electrical activity over a distance tends to equate to zero.

Gavilan and Sanjuan (1964) claimed the first non-surgical recordings of the CM in man using an electrode placed on the surface of the tympanic membrane. They used no electronic averaging equipment so there is some scepticism regarding the results. Irrefutable responses were obtained by Yoshie and Yamaura (1969) using electrodes either embedded in the meatus or placed through the drum on to the promontory. Keidel (1971b) reported a method of recording both SP and CM from electrodes placed on the hard palate. Beagley and Gibson (1976) reported a clinical application of the CM in man for determining whether the site of hearing dysfunction lay in the cochlear or the acoustic nerve, but they found a considerable overlap between the results.

The clinical use of absolute CM measurements is undecided, as much more work is needed before precise information about the function of hair cells can be deduced (Hoke, 1976). A possible clinical application of the CM lies in its use as a relative measure; for instance, Gibson, Ramsden and Moffat (1977) have used CM measurements to show the immediate effects of a vasodilator on the abnormal human cochlea.

The summating potential (SP) is a high threshold DC response characterised by a shift in the baseline of the trace during the period of the stimulus. It was first demonstrated by Davis, Fernández and McAuliffe (1950), who hoped initially that the SP represented the post-synaptic generator potential, but Goldstein (1954) showed this belief was essentially incorrect. Originally, it was thought that the CM were derived mainly from the outer hair cells whilst the SP came from inner hair cells (Davis, 1960), but it has been shown (Stopp and Whitfield, 1964) that SP can be obtained in pigeons even though there are no inner hair cells in the avian cochlea. Davis (1968) later considered the SP as merely an incidental by-product arising from asymmetry in the mechanism that produces the CM rather than as an indication of a major physiological mechanism. This interpretation is probably too simplistic, as recent work (Dallos, Schoeny and Cheatham, 1972) reveals that the SP is a multi-component response arising from more than one source of non-linear electrical activity within the cochlea. The major source is probably linked to cochlear microphonic distortions, but the possibility of a post-synaptic generator potential component is not entirely excluded. The discussions concerning the origins of the SP are continued in Chapter Four.

The other evoked responses

There are many auditory evoked potentials arising from both muscular and neural structures which have not yet been mentioned in this review. Davis (1972) lists the neural responses. The following of these responses seem the most likely to have clinical applications:

The middle latency response (Chapter 8)

Mendel and Goldstein (1969) have investigated low voltage waves with onset latencies of 25–50 ms which are thought to be derived from the medial geniculate and primary cortical projection areas. They found that these early or fast components often seen in CERA recordings were stable during sleep and under anaesthesia (Mendel and Hosick, 1975). They believed that this response might prove better for testing young children than CERA. Davis and Hirsh (1973) investigated forty retarded children but they concluded that they found the fast cortical responses could not always be identified and so they believed that CERA was more reliable. Zerlin, Naunton and Mowry, 1973, managed, however, to obtain more consistent fast responses by using third octave click stimuli.

The frequency-following response

A sound-evoked sinusoidal response can be recorded in man with active electrodes placed in the temporal area of the scalp (Michelson and Vincent, 1975). This response is similar in its characteristics to the *frequency-following response* recorded by Worden and Marsh (1968) in animals. It was first obtained in man by Moushegian, Rupert and Stillman (1973). The response resembles the CM, as it reproduces the electrical waveform of the sound input with an onset latency of approximately 6ms. It appears that it is possible to obtain measurable responses using stimuli only 15–20 dB above the hearing threshold and that these responses are frequency specific. Further work is necessary before it will be known whether the response may be used as a means of assessing hearing acuity and so the method has not been included in this book.

The contingent negative variation (CNV) (Chapter 7)

This response requires the subject to be conditioned to expect the stimulus. It was first described by Walter and his co-workers (1964). The subject is asked to perform a task, such as pressing a switch, every time that he hears a sound. An expectancy wave develops shown by a shift in the baseline of the EEG tracing. The important aspect of this response is that it shows that the sound has been processed by higher cortical areas. Burian, Gestring and Haider (1969) have related the CNV to meaningful words and have suggested that it may be used as an objective test for word discrimination. It would be interesting, obviously, to use this test in the assessment of aphasic children but unfortunately it has proved to be a difficult response to evoke in such cases. The CNV lacks stability when recorded from very young children and subjects with learning and emotional problems (Skinner, 1972).

Acoustically-induced DC potential shifts

Keidel (1971a) has demonstrated another phenomenon similar to the CNV but not requiring conditioning. The response is co-extensive in time with a pure tone stimulus of 1–10 seconds' duration. It may be related to the attentiveness of the subject and so have a future role in audiometry as a means of assessing the higher auditory functions.

Conclusions

An account of the development of the various acoustic electrical responses has been given and some attempt has been made to show the major advantages or disadvantages of each method. Before the availability of averaging techniques, only psychogalvanic skin response audiometry and perhaps electroencephalographic audiometry met with any clinical acceptance and even then the usefulness of such tests was questionable. Following the introduction of the averager, less than twenty years ago, there has been an explosion of interest in ERA and now several very useful methods of assessing the auditory thresholds are available. It is now quite possible to estimate the auditory status of any subject objectively. In older patients, cortical responses indicate adequately the pure tone auditory thresholds. In younger patients, electrocochleography and BER yield a clear picture of the auditory function at a cochlear or brainstem level and myogenic responses may be used to obtain an approximate idea of the hearing status without the need for sedation. More recently, it has become possible to obtain information which helps to locate the actual site of auditory dysfunction and it is hoped that ERA will become a powerful neuro-otological tool.

2. The Apparatus for ERA

The apparatus needed for electric response audiometry is complex and expensive. Unless one is familiar with electronics, the apparatus seems as daunting at first sight as the controls of Concorde. Fortunately, it consists of several components each of which may be discussed separately and which in themselves are not difficult to understand. The clinician need not know the details of the circuits involved but should know the function of each part so that if problems develop during a recording session, he can make arrangements to overcome them. Once the basic principle of each part is understood and one knows how the parts function together, the whole apparatus seems amazingly simple and one soon learns to operate the machine with panache.

Basically, the equipment consists of one part which records the responses (electrodes, amplifiers, filters, averager, display and permanent recording device) and a separate part which provides the necessary sounds to evoke the response (an audiometer which feeds the sounds to a transducer—e.g. a loudspeaker, earphone or bone conductor). One also has to consider the environment in which the testing is performed and any useful pieces of auxilliary equipment needed for checking the apparatus (Fig. 2.1).

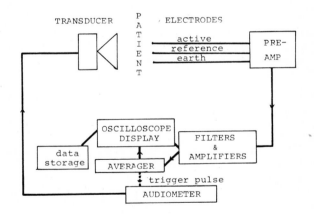

Fig. 2.1 Block diagram of ERA apparatus.

The test environment

There are several important factors to be considered when deciding which position within a hospital or similar building to site the apparatus. Perhaps the first consideration is to have it placed in a convenient room which is readily accessible to those who use it. If the work is to be mainly clinical, it is a great advantage to have the apparatus close to the place where the patients are seen. If children are to be anaesthetised, it is best to have the equipment near the operating theatres and wards so that the anaesthetists do not feel insecure in some inaccessible building. It is most unwise even to contemplate transporting the equipment temporarily into actual operating theatres unless one is prepared to expend a lot of energy and time. Frequent movement of the delicate apparatus will probably result in malfunction and cause knobs to break off and dents to appear. Operating theatres are noisy and contain large pieces of apparatus which produce gross electrical interference, making it very difficult to identify any responses. If one is going to perform a definite experiment in an operating theatre, several hours of preparation are necessary. It is not sensible to consider trundling equipment into the theatre to check a child's hearing before an operating list is to begin. Once a suitable room for the equipment has been found, it is then possible to consider the other important factors. These factors are:

1. *The lay-out of the area.* Sufficient space must be available for the people performing the test, the subject, and the equipment which may include couches, operating microscopes and anaesthetic apparatus. The patient should not be too close to the averaging equipment, as this is usually a source of electrical interference and rather noisy. Since it is pleasant for the operator to be able to talk during the procedure, it is recommended that the patient is positioned in one room whilst the bulk of the apparatus is in another. A window should be available through which the patient may be observed (an alternative is a close-circuit television). When only one room is available, a partition is necessary. At The London Hospital where electrocochleography is mostly performed on co-operative adults, the patients are tested in a room within the out-patient clinic which normally houses an operating microscope, and the main apparatus is placed outside the room in the actual clinic.

2. *Electrical interference.* Hospitals are full of apparatus which produce electrical or other types of interference. Once the ERA apparatus has been installed, it is usually necessary to engage in several hours of detective work tracking each source of interference: transformers emit interference based on 50 hertz (AC mains frequency) and higher harmonics of that frequency. Fluorescent lights within about 15 feet of the electrodes must be disconnected. In some rooms, a ring main may interfere with the apparatus and it may be necessary to place an isolating switch outside the test chamber so that all the mains circuits within that area can be turned off. Generally, the removal of interference from these sources is all that is required. Occasionally, one may be unlucky enough to have some other machinery in the vicinity which has to be suppressed.

In hospitals, 'bleeps' (small single tone paging devices) are a nuisance to the ERA worker. They usually emit a high frequency which may interfere with those tests in which the response frequency lies in the same range. Unless the test room is electrically screened, it is impossible to exclude this interference. Most commercial equipment has a device for rejecting noisy traces before they are included into the averaged response (*See* page 30); by using such a device, it is usually possible to overcome this difficulty. Alternatively, it is possible to construct a unit that receives the 'bleep' transmission and to use that to trigger the signal rejection device.

Finally, it is possible to screen the patient electrically, but under normal circumstances this is not essential. Either the whole room has to be treated, including the doors and lights, or a Faraday cage is needed; it is not very helpful merely to screen one wall.

3. *Acoustic interference.* Ideally all the tests should be conducted within a sound-proofed chamber. Such a chamber is expensive but good examples may be seen at leading ERA centres. It is possible to perform valid clinical work without a sound-proofed area, although there are bound to be some inaccuracies when responses are sought using minimal intensities of stimulation. The usual compromise is to have the test room sound-treated (carpeted, doorways sealed with felt, and windows double glazed). It is also an advantage to conduct the tests using an earphone rather than a loudspeaker. The earphone may be placed inside an acoustically-treated capsule to exclude further extraneous noise. Unfortunately children may not tolerate such a heavy piece of apparatus on their heads. For those centres not lucky enough to have a properly sound-proofed test area, earphones inside acoustically-sealed units provide a very worthwhile alternative.

A further disadvantage of using a loudspeaker is that during free field testing soundwaves will reverberate inside the test room. These echoes may interfere with both the evoked response and the calibration, and if a loudspeaker is to be used accurately, the patient should be tested in an anechoic room.

The stimulating apparatus

It is convenient to consider the apparatus which produces the sound stimulus as a separate entity but it must be remembered that the timing of the onset of the stimulus must be accurately linked to the averager. A *trigger* common to both units is required so that each stimulus occurs at a definite time during each analysis period.

The sound stimulus used has to meet certain requirements depending on the type of response to be averaged. These individual requirements will be discussed in detail in the chapters which deal with each response. The stimulus generator produces first an electrical waveform which is later transduced into the acoustic waveform or stimulus. This electrical waveform is amplified and then passed to a device (an attenuator) which decreases the output by known increments so that the stimulus intensity can be varied in five decibel steps. Finally, the signal is fed to the transducer (usually an earphone or loudspeaker) which changes the electrical waveform into its corresponding acoustic waveform. The accuracy with which this last step is made depends on the quality, and cost, of the transducer. The number of stimuli required and the rate of the presentations is determined by the rate of triggering so that each presentation is synchronised with the sweeps of the averager to allow averaging.

The stimulus

The stimulus itself is of paramount importance for if the input is uncertain, no interpretation of the output (evoked response) can be made. Ideally a stimulus must fulfil three requirements; it must be exact in timing so that the latency of the response is clear, it must be frequency-specific and its intensity must be known.

The earliest recordings were made using simple click stimuli. These are easily produced by sending brief rectangular electrical pulses through a transducer. A click stimulus provides a precise stimulus for timing purposes, and as it stimulates the whole basal portion of the cochlea almost instantaneously, it results in close synchrony of firing of the individual nerve fibres in this area and hence produces a large, clear evoked response. A click stimulus is not frequency-specific as it does, in fact, stimulate the whole of the cochlea.

A frequency-specific stimulus is a pure tone devoid of any click artefacts. Such a stimulus must have a gradual rise and fall time to avoid scattering the acoustic energy. The human brain is unable to make an accurate assessment of frequency unless the pure tone stimulus has a duration of at least 200 milliseconds (ms). Audiometers used for psychophysical measurements usually present stimuli with a rise and fall time of at least 20 ms, but such a stimulus is clearly impractical for ERA, especially when the faster responses (ECochG, BER) are sought. The slow rise time would result in a loss of synchrony as individual nerve fibres would fire at different moments during the rise of the stimulus and this would lead to blurring of the averaged response.

Davis (1976a) summarises the problem well. There is a conflict of stimulus requirements for ERA. On the one hand the stimulus must be brief, and on the other, it needs a long rise time to provide frequency-selectivity. Davis (1976a) cites the Gabor logon theory (1947) which provides a mathematical model of these difficulties. This theory states that if the pure tone stimulus conforms to a Gaussian distribution curve, its rise and fall time can be quantified as its standard deviation. Under these circumstances, the product of minimal Δt (time) and the minimal Δf (frequency) is a constant and so the ideal stimulus can be calculated. In practice, pure tone stimuli are usually shaped to consist of not only a rise and fall but also a plateau of varying lengths so that they do not fulfil the requirements of the theorem.

Click stimuli

The responses with short onset latencies, such as the action potential (AP/E-CochG), brainstem responses (BER), myogenic responses and even the middle latency responses are best evoked by clicks. The fast onset of the click results in good synchronisation of the neural impulses as already discussed.

It is one matter, however, to produce an electrical waveform with a very rapid onset and another to produce a similar acoustic waveform. The transducer cannot react as quickly as an electrical signal as it actually needs to 'vibrate'. The accuracy with which a transducer produces an acoustic signal depends on the quality of its construction. Figure 2.2 shows the electrical input and the acoustic waveform of a click produced by a modestly priced loudspeaker.

A click stimulus stimulates the whole of the cochlea, although the synchronisation of the neural impulses from the more apical regions is poor due to the nature of the travelling wave. Analysis of a typical click stimulus (Fig. 2.3) reveals that it

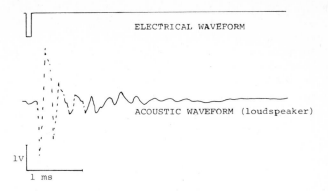

Fig. 2.2 Top line: electrical input to loudspeaker. Bottom line: click acoustic waveform derived from the loudspeaker.

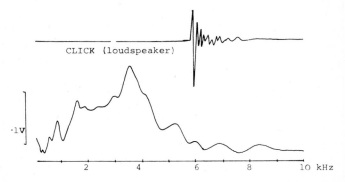

Fig. 2.3 Analysis of a click stimulus. Top line: acoustic waveform. Bottom line: frequency/power spectrum.

contains a wide spectrum of frequencies and that at its onset the higher frequencies predominate. Virtually all acoustic clicks used for ERA have a maximum energy lying between 2–3 kHz. It is possible to present masking noise simultaneously with the click stimulus and, by various techniques (*see* Chapter Four) frequency-specific information can be obtained. Masking is, however, a noisy procedure and it can make threshold estimations difficult. When frequency-specific information is sought, it is more usual to employ a frequency-specific stimulus.

Tonal stimuli

The slow responses such as the cortical responses (CERA and CNV) may be evoked by a tone burst of several milliseconds duration which allows for excellent frequency-specificity. This section concentrates on the tone burst needed for the faster responses.

First, one should consider the acoustic problems. All simple transducers are more resonant to some frequencies than to others and they are seldom critically-damped. Even if a perfect signal is generated electrically, it may be distorted in its acoustic form. There are other acoustic problems which occur before the signal actually reaches the cochlea. The external acoustic meatus has a resonant peak around 4 kHz and the ossicular chain has several resonant peaks which may vary under different conditions; prominent peaks commonly occur at 900 Hz and 1.5 kHz. It is difficult to be sure of the exact waveform which eventually reaches the cochlea. Some workers place minute microphones deep within the external meatus to try to minimise these problems, but it is seldom necessary to go to such lengths for clinical ERA purposes.

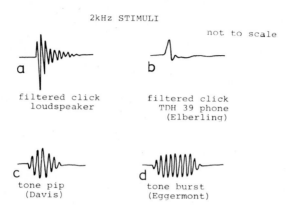

Fig. 2.4 Examples of various transient 2 kHz stimuli.

Filtered clicks (Fig. 2.4a)   A click may be passed through high and low pass filters to eliminate all frequencies except those within a limited bandwidth. Such a procedure may result in a fast rise time electrically which cannot be handled in a frequency-specific manner by the transducer. Analysis of the acoustic waveform, especially that of the onset which actually evokes the response, usually reveals high frequency transients.

Elberling (1976b) describes a method of obtaining frequency–specificity from click–like stimuli. He cleverly selects a transducer which resonates at the desired frequency. He uses a TDH39 earphone to obtain a 2 kHz 'click' and an Audivox 9C earphone to obtain an 8 kHz 'click'. It is not possible to produce such stimuli at frequencies lower than 2 kHz.

Tone pips (Fig. 2.4b)   A more satisfactory method of producing a frequency–specific stimulus involves passing a single sinusoidal wave (rather than a click) which starts and stops at zero crossings through the high and low pass filters. Such a method is employed in the Amplaid Mk III audiometer and other commercially-available equipment.

Tone bursts (Fig. 2.4c)   Longer duration stimuli may be produced by passing more than one sinusoidal wave through the high and low pass filters. Alternatively, stimuli can be shaped by gating pure tone stimuli with linear ramps. Eggermont and Spoor (1973a) used tone bursts which had two periods of sine waves during the rise and fall and a plateau of six periods. This wave envelope has a duration which is very dependent on the frequency of the stimulus—low frequency tone bursts last several milliseconds. Unfortunately it is not safe to shorten the period of the stimulus onset as rise times of less than two cycles may, at high intensities, produce a high frequency transient capable of evoking a response.

Masking noise. A masking noise is a sound containing a range of frequencies (either a wide range or a narrow range centred on some particular frequency) and may be used to prevent the hearing of a sound or part of a sound. In conventional audiometry, masking is generally employed to prevent the non-stimulated ear from hearing the stimulus delivered to the ear under test—i.e. to prevent cross-talk. A great advantage of electrocochleography is that no masking of the opposite ear is required, but for all later responses masking is essential. This is especially true when bone conduction thresholds are sought. Generally, it is best to use narrow band masking centred on the frequency of the stimulus.

Masking may also be used to obtain frequency-specific information. The principle of successive high pass masking was first described by Teas, Eldredge and Davis (1962). Eggermont and Odenthal (1974a) used selective masking to obtain low frequency information using transtympanic electrocochleography. Further details are given in Chapter 4.

The amplifier

Once formed, the electrical waveform is amplified. This is a relatively straightforward matter accepting that the amplifier must be of sufficient quality not to cause distortion.

The attenuator

Clinically it is essential to be able to present the stimulus at varying intensities. This is usually achieved by attenuating the input and the output of the power amplifier. It is often arranged in 5-decibel steps.

Calibration

Accurate calibration of the intensity of the stimulus that actually reaches the tympanic membrane is essential if precise work is to be performed. This calibration may be achieved either by using a sound pressure level meter (SPL), using a biological standard (HL) or by comparing the acoustic waveform of the stimulus with a known calibrated signal on an oscilloscope. (Peak equivalent SPL). It is a comparatively simple affair to calibrate a pure tone stimulus lasting several milliseconds but far more difficult to do so with transient stimuli such as clicks.

The sound pressure level (SPL) weighting curves.

These are derived from physical measurements, conveniently measured in decibels. Decibels form a logarithmic scale based on the ratio of the root mean square (rms) sound pressure and a reference sound pressure level. The threshold of hearing, for a sound of given character, is the minimum value of the rms sound pressure which excites the sensation of hearing. Several sound pressure level weighting curves have been designed (Appendix 2) to reflect the thresholds of normal hearing. At the upper and lower frequencies of the human auditory range, a greater sound pressure is required to reach the psychophysical thresh-old. In the weighting curves A, B, C and D, the reference level of 0 dB at 1000 hertz is a sound pressure of $20\,\mu P$ (0.0002 dynes/cm²). The advantage of using these scales is that they are physical measures which can be made using a sound pressure level meter. When clicks are to be calibrated, there are problems, since even the most sophisticated sound level meter will not react in time to a transient stimulus. Whilst an impulse sound level meter may be reasonably accurate with tone bursts even this will fail in the case of abrupt clicks.

Peak equivalent SPL.

To overcome the problem of measurement outlined in the previous paragraph, some workers compare the maximum amplitude of the signal to be calibrated with that of a known signal using an oscilloscope. Again there are problems when calibrating clicks. The main difficulty is due to temporal summation. Temporal auditory summation is the physiological process by which the intensity required to reach the psychophysical threshold for a tone increases as the duration of the tone is decreased (Wright, 1968). A stimulus of one millisecond duration requires approximately 20 dB greater intensity than the same stimulus presented over one second in order to be heard. Thus, peak equivalent measurements may be accurate but in the case of transient stimuli they will not relate very closely to the dB scales with which the clinician is familiar.

Biological calibration.

Most clinical audiometers are calibrated using a biological scale, usually the International Standard Reference Zero (ISO) recommendation R389. 0 dB refers to the threshold of hearing at the specified frequency using a specified type of earphone, the modal value being determined by testing an adequately large number of ears of otologically normal subjects within the age limits of 18–24 years inclusive, an otologically normal subject being a person in a normal state of health who is free from all signs or symptoms of ear disease and from wax in the ear canal and who has no history of noise exposure.

Biological calibration is the most convenient means of calibrating the transient stimuli used in ERA. One merely finds a number of young 'volunteers' and sets the machine to zero (0 dB HL). There are, of course, some problems. Patients with auditory disorders often do not show the normal amounts of temporal auditory summation and so in their cases the calibration is difficult. Responses obtained at cochlear level may not be prone to temporal auditory summation and so, in theory at least, it is possible that the cochlea reacts to a stimulus that the brain does not detect. One consolation is that the loudness function of clicks does not appear to differ significantly from pure tones (Cazals and Stephens, 1975).

The human brain is unable to determine the frequency or pitch of a tonal stimulus accurately unless the stimulus is presented for a duration of more than 200 milliseconds. For stimuli lasting less than 5 milliseconds, pitch judgement is absent (Whitfield, 1956). Although it may not be possible to determine the pitch of these transient stimuli subjectively, it is more than likely that they still stimulate the cochlea in a frequency-specific manner. The effect of the repetition rate of the stimulus presentation on the psychophysical threshold is minimal (Garner, 1947) and can in practice be discounted.

The time taken for the stimulus to reach the ears

Sound travels relatively slowly through air and takes four seconds to travel a mile, which is slower than many aircraft today. It takes approximately one millisecond for sound to travel one foot. One may therefore expect the latency of an evoked response to be 3 ms later when evoked by a loudspeaker placed a meter from the ear than when the same stimulus is delivered by an earphone. If accurate latency records are to be made, it is important always to know the timing of the sound as it reaches the tympanic membrane. This is easily discovered by using a microphone placed at the equivalent distance.

The attenuation of sound with distance

A simple guide is that when one doubles the distance from the sound source, the sound intensity is reduced by 6 dB. This illustrates the importance of always placing the loudspeaker at exactly the same distance from the ear. (When a rather questionable response has been obtained at the maximum output of the audiometer, a quite useful technique is to decrease the loudspeaker distance from the calibrated position; if one halves and then halves again the distance, approximately 12 dB is added to the maximum output intensity).

The recording apparatus

Assuming that a bio-electric response has been evoked as a result of the stimulus, it must then be collected and recorded. The recording apparatus consists of the electrodes, amplifiers, filters, averager and display, together with some device for obtaining a permanent record.

The electrodes

The form of the electrode varies according to the position where it has to be placed on the subject. In simplest terms, the electrodes used for ERA may be either 'surface' or 'specialised'. Most commonly monopolar recordings are taken. An active electrode (usually tagged red) is placed nearest the source of potential. A reference electrode (usually tagged black) is placed at a neutral point such as the earlobe in trans-tympanic ECochG. The earth electrode (usually tagged green) is placed at a further neutral point (commonly the forehead). Monopolar or common reference recordings compare the output of the active and earth electrode with that of the reference electrode. This method is best for the recording of evoked potentials and less liable to produce distortions than bipolar recordings. Several methods of ERA including the cortical and brainstem responses are really 'dipolar' recordings, the reference electrode not being passive but contributing to the response.

Surface electrodes. Since the electrode is to be placed on the skin, it is possible to take measures to reduce the skin to electrode resistance to a minimum and gain the best conditions for interference-free recordings. The most commonly used electrodes are the standard silver/silver chloride EEG disc variety (Fig. 2.5). The layer of silver chloride appears almost black on the surface of the electrode and helps to decrease its polarisation when placed on the skin. After being used many times, the silver chloride wears off and the electrode appears silver. At this stage it is wise to replace the silver chloride by using the electrode as an anode and electrolyse a solution of salt. If in doubt one can usually find a friendly EEG technician who may be bribed to chloride one's electrodes!

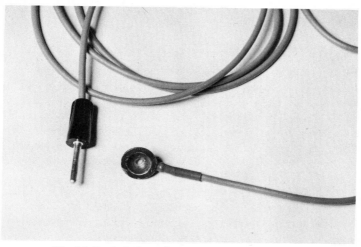

Fig. 2.5 Typical silver/silver chloride disc electrode.

Before applying the electrode to the skin, it is helpful to remove any grease or make-up on the skin with acetone solution. The electrode is fixed in position with either an adhesive disc, or quick drying glue, or both. Next the inside of the electrode or dome is *completely* filled with high conductivity electrode gel so that it exudes through the hole in the top of the dome. The surface of the underlying skin can be abraided with a blunt needle to reduce the resistance further. Finally the resistance between pairs of surface electrodes is checked to make sure the system functions. A multimeter may be used to measure the resistance to current flowing and a resistance reading of less than 5 kΩ (kilo-ohms) generally is acceptable. The trans-tympanic electrode used for electrocochleography has a very high input impedance (about 60 kΩ) so it is not necessary to reduce the resistance of the reference and earth electrodes to low levels in this instance. Sometimes the patient may feel current from the multimeter flowing, or occasionally the current may polarize the electrodes, one becoming an anode and the other a cathode as in electrolysis; this results in their becoming coated and increases their resistance. This is simply prevented by briefly reversing polarities. It is not safe to use a multimeter to check the resistance of a transtympanic electrode so the impedance is usually measured using an impedance measuring device which relies on an alternating low level current. Such a device is very useful when the electrocochleogram is used over periods of time to monitor possible changes in the potentials (e.g. after drug infusions).

Specialised electrodes. Some responses, such as electrocochleography, require a special electrode that may be placed in a particular anatomical position (either through the tympanic membrane or on it). The transtympanic electrode is usually a thin needle insulated except at its very tip. The tympanic electrode is usually a silver ball electrode which may be coated with silver chloride. It is wise to check the integrity of these electrodes carefully before they are inserted into the patient's ear. One lead of the multimeter can be connected to the lead of the active electrode whilst the other is attached to a piece of sterile metal foil. When the tip of the electrode touches the foil, current should flow with no measurable resistance.

The pre-amplifier

This is usually placed close to the electrodes so that the signal may be amplified before it is sent down cables to reach the main bulk of the recording equipment which is commonly sited in another room. The evoked response is minute, measuring only a few millionths of a volt, and if this were to travel far it could easily be swamped by interference. Therefore the signal is amplified, perhaps a hundred times, so that it is large compared with any incidental electrical activity picked up later. Two other features of the pre-amplifier are important; the common mode rejection and the input impedance.

Common mode rejection is the rejection of any signal which is the same or common to both the active and the reference electrode. For example, both these electrodes pick up mains interference to almost the same extent, and by rejecting the common signal the problem is virtually overcome.

Input impedance may be simply considered as the amount of electricity which may flow into the system. If the electrode resistance is high as in transtympanic electrocochleography, the electrodes will limit the amount of electrical signal flowing to the pre-amplifier. It would be dangerous therefore to have an input impedance lower than the electrode resistance, as this would not only accommodate the signal flowing in but also leave 'the gate open' for other sources of electricity. Ideally one should have an input impedance which matches exactly the resistance of the electrodes. In practice, it is best to have an input impedance which is always higher than the electrode resistance, as this effectively 'closes the gate' for the admission of extraneous electrical interference.

The main amplifier

The final amplification or *gain* is usually achieved by an amplifier actually sited on the main bulk of the recording apparatus. This is convenient, as the gain may be altered without having to keep walking into the test area each time. An important feature of both the pre-amplifier and especially of the main amplifier is that they accurately amplify all the frequencies in the physiological spectrum without distortion (biological amplification). The amount of amplification used must be known accurately. This is usually achieved by feeding a signal of a known size (e.g. $10 \mu V$) into the pre-amplifier. The Madsen equipment has a facility for automatic gain control and provision has been made for a calibration signal to be averaged simultaneously with every ERA response obtained.

Filters

The amplified signal from the patient will contain a wide spectrum of frequencies which is limited only by the characteristics of the amplifier itself. Each response in ERA has a particular range of frequencies within which the energy lies. If one knows this range, it is possible to exclude all the other frequencies which are not adding to the response but form only a source of artefactual contamination. For instance, the energy of the slow cortical responses lie chiefly in the range of 4–6 Hz. It is therefore worthwhile to place a high pass filter (below which frequency nothing passes) at 1.6 Hz and a low pass filter (above which frequency nothing passes) at 13 Hz. The specific filters for the other responses will be discussed in the relevant chapters.

The situation, however, is not quite so simple as it seems, because no filter can be so abrupt as to cut off at exactly the frequency stated. This 'roll-off' or 'cut-off' capability is usually measured in dB per octave. ENT surgeons, not familiar with electronics, may find it easier to consider the effect of a 512 Hz low-pass filter with 20 dB 'roll-off' by imagining a pure tone audiogram. Low-pass implies that only frequencies below 512 Hz can pass freely. At each octave (1024, 2048, 4096 Hz etc.) above 512 Hz, 20 dB less energy can pass. A sharp filter would have a roll-off of perhaps 60 dB per octave whilst a more gradual filter might have a roll-off of only 10 dB per octave. Obviously the sharper the filtering, the less the power from the unwanted frequencies which is being accepted for averaging. However, if a filter is made too sharp, it may distort the signal and produce an artefact.

The unaveraged signal

It is advantageous to incorporate a facility for examining the unaveraged signal both before and during the test procedure. One soon learns to recognise the pattern of an acceptable signal and to detect certain problems that may ruin the recordings.

Artefact rejection

One of the most frustrating sights during an ERA procedure is to watch an averaged response slowly building only to be suddenly swamped by an artefact. Artefacts may be serious because they can be unwittingly accepted as true evoked responses and there are many cases in which deaf children have been falsely labelled as hearing. So important is the problem of artefacts that virtually every established worker has a method of recognising and rejecting them. These methods may either be 'on-line' or coincidental with the recording or 'off-line' when the recording is processed after the recording session.

Off-line methods are not very practicable clinically as they involve time. The recording is examined and the epochs during averaging when artefacts occurred are noted. The recording is then altered in such a way as to prevent these epochs from averaging. Templates of true responses may be constructed so that any epoch which contains a waveform differing from the template by a specified amount is identified and excluded.

On-line methods.   These methods are far more practicable, as little extra time is added to the test procedure. There are manual and automatic systems. Manual systems comprise simply a switch which can be moved whenever an artefact is recognised on the on-going trace. This technique is invaluable to counter

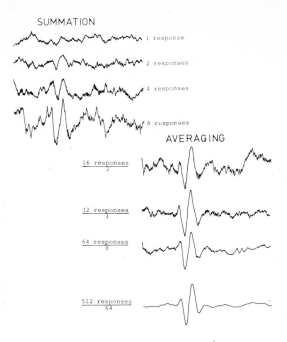

Fig. 2.6 An illustration of the summation and averaging techniques used for ERA.

hospital 'bleep' signals. The switch must not simply stop the averager in the middle of an epoch but has to be arranged either to prevent further epochs from being accepted or, preferably, prevent the actual epoch and its immediate predecessors from being passed from a memory into the averager.

Automatic systems of artefact recognition and rejection are of great value, especially in those tests in which an attempt is being made to average a response from a young active subject. The recognition of an artefact may be incredibly sophisticated and computerised. Alternatively, rejection may be based on a simple device which merely detects any signal that exceeds certain preset voltage limits. Once an artefact has been recognised, steps must be taken to prevent that epoch from entering the averager. Usually this is done by delaying the epoch in a memory store until the monitoring has been completed. Then, if it contains an artefact, it is cleared without passing forward to the averager

The averager

This is the heart of the entire system. The simple theory is that the response always occurs at a definite time after the stimulus and so occurs at a definite point during each epoch or sweep presented to the averager. It is, however, hidden to a greater or lesser extent by random potentials from various sources. If each epoch is added to the next, the response being time-locked grows steadily whilst the random activity tends to cancel itself (Fig. 2.6a). A selected number of responses can be summated in this way. The final result may be divided by a known factor, so reducing both the size of the response and the other fluctuations on the tracing. This makes the final recording clearer (Fig. 2.6b). A more detailed explanation follows.

The theory of operation.   When a repetitive waveform is sampled regularly at a time (t) after its origin, the instantaneous value will be constant. Therefore the average (achieved by dividing the amplitude of the response by a number equal to the number of samples) will be equal to the instantaneous value. When a random waveform, not related to any timing, is sampled regularly, the instantaneous value will differ and may be of either polarity. Thus, after a number of samples have been averaged, the value will be asymptotic to zero. Any noise must not be harmonically related to the stimulus rate. Equipment, such as the Medelec apparatus, has a facility for randomising the triggering to aid the solution to this problem should it arise.

The mathematical theory of operation.   The principle underlying the extraction of a signal from noise by summating techniques may be analysed mathematically. It is quite simple to calculate that the amplitude of a synchronised response (A) increases in direct proportion to the number of summations (N) by:

$$\sum_{i=1}^{N} A_i = A_1 + A_2 + A_3 \ldots \ldots A_N = N \cdot A$$

The noise (B) will add up according to the rms values:

$$\sqrt{\sum_{i=1}^{N} B_i^2} = \sqrt{B_1^2 + B_2^2 + B_3^2 + \ldots \ldots B_N^2} = B \cdot \sqrt{N}$$

So by combining these equations, the signal to noise ratio may be calculated:

$$\frac{\sum_{i=1}^{N} A_i}{\sqrt{\sum_{i=1}^{N} B_i^2}} = \frac{N \cdot A}{B \cdot \sqrt{N}} = \sqrt{N} \cdot \frac{A}{B}$$

The signal to noise ratio has therefore been improved by the square root of N. Theoretically it would be possible to infinitely improve the signal to noise ratio, but in practice this is not possible since the biological response patterns are somewhat variable. The timing of the response to the stimulus may alter (time jitter) and as a result the averaged response may eventually become broadened and decreased in amplitude.

Computing facilities

Depending on the sophistication (and unfortunately the expense) of the equipment, facilities can be provided for analysing and performing mathematical functions with the response obtained. It is useful to have provision for measuring accurately the timing or latency of each response and for measuring its size or amplitude. It may also be helpful to be able to invert individual responses or to be able to add and subtract them from another. Examples of the clinical use of subtracting one response from another are given in the chapter on electrocochleography (Chapter 4).

Display

It is important to be able to examine the results of averaging at the time of testing and before a permanent record is taken. Most apparatus displays this information on an oscilloscope. There is, also, an advantage to being able actually to see each response building during averaging. One can often spot the sudden baseline fluctuations which occur when a large transient artefact contaminates the response. This option is especially helpful when one is trying to detect a response close to the threshold. Most apparatus includes a facility so that measurements of the latency and amplitude of the evoked response can be taken directly from the display.

Latency measurements can be vital in determining the validity of a response by predicting its latency from the previous averaged responses. Latency measurements include peak onset latencies, inter-peak latencies and peak width measurements. The onset latencies are generally useful and may provide evidence of recruitment. Inter-peak latencies are important for the neurological application of BER as they may be used to predict the presence of a lesion between the brainstem nuclei. Peak width measurements are made in ECochG to determine broadening of the combined action potential and summating potential (AP/SP) in certain pathological conditions.

Amplitude measurements are not so important during the actual test period. It is usually quite obvious if a response is larger than expected without the need for any accurate measurement. Amplitude measurements are useful when subsequent analysis of the tracings is undertaken, as they may help to reveal a recruiting hearing loss or other types of dysfunction.

Data storage

Permanent recording facilities

It is an obvious requirement that the data obtained during ERA procedures should be stored for later analysis. This storage may be achieved either by using the memory of a computer, tape, or more simply by making permanent copies of the recording. Permanent records of the averager display may be of two types; pen recordings and photographic prints.

Storage of raw data. The electrical activity recorded from the patient may be recorded on to a magnetic tape or 'floppy-disc'. This data can then be fed into the averager at a later date. The advantage of storing the raw data, rather than the final averaged response, is that manipulations can be accomplished at a later date without inconveniencing the patient. For example, one can feed the raw data through different filter settings to find out how the recording bandwidth alters the shape of the averaged response.

Pen recordings are usually provided by the so-called 'X-Y' plotter. This name results from the horizontal (X) axis and the vertical (Y) axis which govern the passage of the recording pen across the paper. The main advantages are that a clear permanent trace is obtained which may be easily changed in amplitude. The recording may be made directly on to graph paper which simplifies any analysis. The main disadvantages are that the calibration has to be carefully and frequently checked and that each of the recordings takes several seconds to be completed.

Photographic methods usually involve photographing the response as it is displayed on an oscilloscope. The obvious advantage of this method is speed, since each recording is made by simply pressing a button. The photographic film may either be developed later or more usually it is of a rapid self-developing nature (e.g. polaroid). One disadvantage of using such paper is that unless steps are taken to 'fix' the print, further exposure to light will eventually fog the picture. When such a recording is taken, it is sensible to record a timing and an amplitude calibration pulse so that the responses can be properly analysed if one wishes at a later date.

Storage of data must be arranged in such a way that previous work may be readily retrieved. It can be most frustrating to be faced with unlabelled data. Each set of data must be labelled with the patient's name, age, hospital number or address, and the date of testing. The ear which is being tested must be clearly shown. For every response, it must be possible to determine retrospectively the stimulus that evoked it. Apart from the intensity and frequency, details of the stimulus envelope (rise time, plateau and decay) should be known. The amplitude of the averaged response depends on several factors such as the ratio of the number of responses summed to the number of averages (divisions) made. The gain of the amplifiers and the filter settings are noted especially if they are altered during the recording session.

The roll or folder of data should then be stored in a manner which allows quick retrieval. Apart from this measure, it is customary to keep a separate record of the findings in book form. This is both for safety and as a means of quickly checking cases; for example, if the diagnosis is always noted, one can later search the book for the cases of any particular disease, saving the chore of reading through sets of hospital notes. It helps to use a pro forma for noting essential medical points in each case, as far too often hospital notes are lost—especially when the case is of interest!

Conclusions

This chapter has only attempted to give elementary details of the basic theory behind each component part of typical ERA equipment. Further details of the apparatus and gain and filter settings required for obtaining specific responses are given in the relevant chapters under the heading of apparatus. For those workers using the Medelec equipment, typical switch positions for obtaining each response are given in Appendix 3 and this may provide a useful check-list before a patient is actually tested.

3. Cortical Electric Response Audiometry (CERA)—The Slow 'Vertex' Potential

Until a few years ago, the 'slow' cortical response or vertex potential formed the mainstay of electric response audiometry and it was generally understood that unless one clearly stated that some other response was being employed, the term ERA implied the use of this response. The initial enthusiasm that greeted the response has now waned. This is due both to the attraction of the faster responses such as ECochG and BER which are easier to interpret and to some as yet unsolved problems in the use of CERA in testing young children. Nevertheless the slow CERA potential does allow accurate threshold predictions through the entire speech frequency range in adults and older children, and if the answers can be found to the remaining problems, it is probable that this response will once again gain favour.

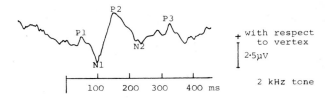

Fig. 3.1 A typical adult response.

Terminology

The typical adult response (Fig. 3.1) shows a small inconsistent positive peak (P1) at 50–75 milliseconds (ms), a large negative peak (N1) at about 100–150 ms and a large positive peak (P2) at about 175–200 ms. The polarity in each case refers to the vertex electrode with respect to the mastoid. Usually this is followed by a low second negative peak (N2) at 200–250 ms which is inconsistent in the adult but may be very prominent in young children, in whom the latency is often even longer. A slow positive wave then follows at about 300 ms which has been associated with the CNV but recent work has shown that it has a different scalp distribution to the CNV and is not affected by the presence of a warning signal (Donchin *et al.*, 1975). This series of electrical waves can be labelled according to their polarity and latency: P50, N100, P200, N250 and P300, but if one wishes to refer to the entire response complex, a simpler term is obviously advantageous. The term 'electroencephalic response audiometry' (ERA) is unsatisfactory nowadays as it is always confused with electric response audiometry (ERA). A few years ago this was often accepted, for the reasons already stated, but today there are a host of different responses used for ERA. For historical reasons, it seems reasonable to use the term 'cortical electric response audiometry' (CERA) as this can be easily accepted by those workers who liked the term ERA to apply only to these responses. There are, however, other responses derived from the cortex of the brain which are used for audiometry, namely, the middle latency responses described by Mendel and Goldstein (1969) which are described in Chapter Eight, and the CNV described in Chapter 7. Davis (1971) suggested firstly that one should label the responses according to their polarity and latency and secondly that cortical responses could be classified as 'early' or 'fast' when occurring before 50 ms, 'slow' when occurring between 50–300 ms, and 'very slow' or 'late' if continuing after 300 ms (e.g. CNV). Alternatively, Bancaud, Bloch and Paillard (1953) and Gastaut (1953) suggested the term 'V' potential (vertex potential), as the anatomical distribution of the slow CERA potential is centred around the vertex. This book uses the term CERA to imply the slow (vertex) potential unless it is stated otherwise.

The history of CERA has been dealt with extensively in Chapter 1 and is not discussed further here.

The anatomy and physiology

The neural auditory pathway leads from the cochlea along the eighth nerve to the brainstem and then passes through various stations within the mid-brain (described in Chapter Five) to reach the medial geniculate body, which is functionally part of the thalamus. Its main output is to the primary cortical areas. Chang (1950) first demonstrated the presence of reverberating neuronal circuits between the medial geniculate body and the cortex.

The boundaries of the auditory cortex cannot be unequivocally stated even in amimals. In man, it is common knowledge that the cortex is far more complicated than in animals. Thus it is inevitable that the exact extent and position of the auditory cortex in man remains a matter for conjecture. There are several possible methods of defining the limits of the auditory cortex. Firstly, the examination of the histological structure of the cortex (Campbell, 1905; Rose, 1949) but present knowledge of the correlation between histological detail and function is too limited to allow accurate localisation of the auditory area. Secondly, one may examine the neural connections. Those parts of the cortex connected directly with the lower auditory centres may be called 'primary areas'. Secondary areas are connected to these primary areas and, in turn, tertiary areas connect with secondary areas, and so on. Unfortunately the situation is not clear-cut: Kiang (1955) and Downman, Woolsey and Lende (1960) have shown that not all the activation of secondary areas is via a primary area, and to confuse matters even more, it has been shown that primary areas may also act as secondary areas, etc. Thirdly, one may examine the electrical potentials in response to acoustic stimulation of the cochlea or electrical stimulation of some part of the lower auditory tract. If the slow wave response is studied, it appears not to be well localised to any area and so gives little indication of the extent of the auditory area. If single unit activity is studied, this is so well localised that thousands of units must be examined before any conclusions are possible. The last possible method is to ablate areas of the cortex and then to examine the animal by behavioural methods. As behavioural responses involve motor as well as sensory mechanisms, this method does not provide a selective basis for such a study.

The only conclusions that can really be drawn from the studies to date in man are that part of the primary auditory area lies in the superior temporal gyrus and that this extends into the transverse temporal gyri, lying on the floor of the posterior ramus of the lateral sulcus behind the insula. It is still a matter for dispute whether the insula and other temporal gyri are primary or secondary areas. The full extent of the secondary areas is not known but it seems likely that areas of the parietal and frontal lobes are involved.

The first cortical responses in man are recorded with an onset latency of 10–30 ms (Celesia *et al.*, 1968). It seems likely that these responses are in fact the middle latency responses reported by Mendel and Goldstein (1969). The CERA responses cannot be primary responses in the sense of being the first response of the cortical cells connected directly to the lower centres, but some evidence suggests (Vaughan, 1969) that these potentials do arise from primary cortical projection areas of the cortex; the delay is either due to reverberating circuits between the medial geniculate body and cortex, or it is due to secondary, tertiary and later responses occurring within the primary area. On the other hand, David and Sohmer (1972) placed electrodes directly on the exposed cortex of the cat, and described a diffuse response arising from a widespread non-primary cortical

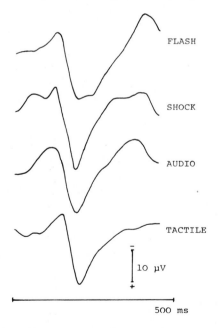

Fig. 3.2 Cortical responses to flash, shock, auditory and tactile stimuli (adapted from Davis *et al.* (1972)).

area, and resembling the human CERA potential. This particular work also suggested that the response was initiated by activity passing up the classical ascending auditory pathways rather than by some alternative route possibly involving the reticular system, but many workers remain unconvinced (Salomon, 1976).

Some characteristics of the slow response

The stimulus modality

Slow responses from the region of the vertex may be evoked by stimulating virtually any sensory input to the brain. Figure 3.2 shows examples of slow responses to flash, shock, auditory and tactile stimuli. The waveform of the slow response differs only in minor details amongst these sensory modalities. Walter (1964) found that the largest amplitude occurred using auditory stimuli. Vaughan (1969) and more recently Davis et al. (1972) have shown that each of the slow responses is derived from the primary cortical projection area of the sensory modality concerned.

The possibility of a tactile modality must be remembered when CERA is used to investigate a deaf subject, especially when a low stimulus frequency is employed. A response to a 500 Hz stimulus, for example, at 110 dB does not necessarily imply that the subject has heard the stimulus, as the vibration produced by such a stimulus can be clearly felt.

The tactile slow response is helpful during CERA procedures in establishing a baseline response. If a subject is tested and no auditory responses are obtained, one is forced either to the conclusion that the subject is deaf or that the apparatus is faulty. If, in the same subject, a clear tactile response is obtained, perhaps by applying a vibrator to the fingertips, then the diagnosis of severe hearing loss is reached with increased reliability.

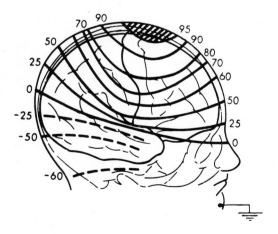

Fig. 3.3 Isopotential map of the slow auditory response (P200) using a chin reference. (Vaughan, H.G. (1969), by permission N.A.S.A.)

Topography of the response

Vaughan (1969) has constructed an isopotential map of the auditory slow response (P200) which is shown in Figure 3.3. The reference electrode was placed on the chin. He used a binaural stimulus of 1 kHz tones at 60 dB SL and he found that the response was absent along a line which roughly represented the surface markings of the Sylvian fissure. The polarity of the response altered as this line was crossed. The maximum response amplitude was recorded from an area on and slightly in front of the vertex of the scalp (rather like the area covered by a skull-cap worn forwards on the head). He concluded from these results that the P200 wave was generated from sources located within the primary auditory projection areas. A similar study of the P300 wave suggested that this potential was derived from a much wider area of the cortex involving the parietal association cortex.

Despite Vaughan's work (1969), there is still disagreement, especially as later workers were unable to confirm his findings (Kooi, Tipton and Marshall, 1971), and a recent article by Picton *et al.* (1974) states that the N1, P2, N2 (50–300 ms) components of the slow auditory response represent a widespread activation of the frontal cortex. It should be remembered, however, that the finding that the responses are generated from within the area encompassed by the primary cortical projections does not necessarily exclude the possibility that the response is of a secondary (or later) nature.

The choice of the electrode sites for recording the slow response is influenced by these findings. Virtually every laboratory places the active electrode either on the vertex or slightly forward of the vertex, and a reference electrode on the mastoid.

The frequency range of the response

The main spectral energy of the slow response is concentrated within the frequency range of 4–6 Hz. It is possible, therefore, to use quite narrow bandpass filtering which helps to exclude disturbances caused by the mains power frequency (50 Hz) and some of the muscle artefacts. Johannsen (1971) investigated the filtering of the slow response and has suggested that the optimum filter settings are 1.6 Hz HPF to 13.6 LPF. He found unexpectedly that the use of a low cut-off frequency of 1.6 Hz enhanced the amplitude of the response. Workers using the Medelec equipment are advised to use a HPF setting of 100 ms (1.6 Hz) and a LPF setting of 10 ms (16 Hz).

The mechanism of the response

It is often assumed that the slow response consists of an additive contribution to the spontaneous EEG activity. Sayers, Beagley and Henshall (1974) have shown this to be incorrect and they believe that the response is mainly due to a reorganisation or constraint of the phase spectra of the existing spontaneous activity of the EEG. They hoped that closer attention to phase characteristics would prove helpful in recognising the response pattern amongst the background noise.

Stimulus characteristics

Intensity.   There are many reports detailing the effect of altering the stimulus intensity on the functions of the slow responses· (Suzuki and Taguchi, 1965; Keidel and Spreng, 1965; Rapin *et al.*, 1965; Rose and Ruhm, 1966; Davis and Zerlin, 1966; Beagley and Knight, 1967; *inter alia*). Each investigator has reported that as the stimulus intensity increases, the peak amplitude of each component increases whilst the latency becomes shorter. Rapin *et al.* (1965) found that the change of latency with alteration of intensity using click stimuli was minimal. At intensities over 60 dB SL, the amplitude of the slow response decreases when using fast stimulus repetition rates. Antinoro, Skinner and Jones (1969) have shown that the relation between stimulus intensity (in dB) and the amplitude (in μV) is linear for low and middle frequencies; this finding can help the prediction of threshold (Skinner, Antinoro and Shimota., 1974). Arlinger (1976a) has also constructed a mathematical model for the extrapolation of threshold using the latency properties of the slow response.

Stimulus frequency.   There appears to be significant interaction between the amplitude of the slow response and the frequency of the stimulus (Antinoro and Skinner, 1968; Antinoro *et al.*, 1969; Rothman, 1970). At equal sensation levels, there appears to be little difference in the amplitude of the response to 250, 500 and 1000 Hz signals but the amplitude does decrease by approximately 20 per cent per octave for frequencies over 1000 Hz.

Stimulus duration.   It is well known that stimulus duration is related to perceived loudness. This phenomenon, known as temporal auditory summation, is the physiological process by which the intensity required to obtain the psychophysical threshold for a tone increases as the duration of the tone is decreased (Wright, 1968). The first mathematical model and equivalent electrical circuit for this event was advanced by Munson (1947). More recently, Zwislocki (1960) has shown that the threshold at 1000 Hz improves by 10 dB for a ten-fold increase in duration up to 200 milliseconds.

It has been reported that the slow response does not reflect temporal summation (Skinner and Jones, 1968; Onishi and Davis, 1968). They reported a slight tendency for the amplitude to increase with signal durations up to 25–50 ms but found no further increase in amplitude using signal durations up to 150 ms. Hyde (1976), on the other hand, has shown convincingly that temporal intergration does occur using signal durations of less than 40 ms. Spreng (1969), however, believes that this finding is due to an overlapping effect between the on and off activity of the response. He reported that, using soft switched (1/3 octave filtered) sinusoidal tones, there was augmentation of nearly all components with increasing signal duration in the range of 3–300 ms.

Despite the report by Spreng (1969), most workers accept that the slow response is predominantly an on-effect and use a stimulus duration of 25–50 ms as this is sufficiently long to allow accurate frequency determination without causing a significant decline in amplitude.

Stimulus rise time.   Onishi and Davis (1968) found that the amplitude of the slow response components (N100, P200) diminished only very gradually with an increase in the rise time of the stimulus up to 30 ms, but after 30 ms a more distinctive amplitude reduction occurred. Skinner and Jones (1968) reported similar findings but found the amplitude reduction began to be marked after

25 ms. No interaction between sensation level and rise time from 30–90 dB SL was reported. It is probable that a rise time of 25–30 ms is optimum because it is gradual enough to avoid click artefacts and sufficiently abrupt to evoke a clear response.

Influence of stimulus repetition rate. Davis *et al.* (1966) reported that the slow response took approximately 10 seconds to recover after each stimulus before it could be evoked fully again. Keidel and Spreng (1965) found that further small increases in amplitude occurred up to about 30 seconds. The amplitude of the N100, P200 complex is diminished, therefore, when the stimulus repetition rate is fast.

The smallest number of responses which must be averaged to produce adequate resolution at low stimulus intensities is reported as 32 (Davis *et al.*, 1966) but most other workers have averaged at least 50 responses (Leibman and Graham, 1967). Although the maximum response amplitude occurs using a stimulus presentation rate of one every 10 seconds or more, this would obviously prolong the procedure to such an extent that it would hardly be practicable. Most workers use a presentation rate of between one each 1–2 seconds for clinical purposes.

Regular versus irregular stimulus repetition rates. It is found that if an irregular (random) stimulus repetition rate is used, the amplitude of the response is consistently larger (Tyberghein and Forrez, 1969). Randomisation of the stimulus application aids the averager in suppressing any regular source of interference, such as the EEG alpha rhythm and may help by increasing the attention of the subject.

The evoking factor of the stimulus. It is widely accepted that the slow response contains components related both to the onset and continuation of the stimulus ('on-response') and to the switching off of the stimulus ('off-response') (Davis and Zerlin, 1966). Spreng (1969), as already stated, has warned that short duration stimulation will lead to a superimposition of these two response types. The 'on-response' is the predominant activity when short duration stimuli are used; this is partly due to the slow recovery period of the response.

Binaural versus monaural stimulation. The amplitude of the response is enhanced if the stimulus is presented to both ears simultaneously. This finding correlates well with the psycho-acoustical finding of an apparent increase in loudness on binaural stimulation.

Contralateral masking. The amplitude of the slow response to a left ear stimulus is the same, allowing for subject variability, regardless of whether the recording is made from the right side of the head or the left. It is not possible to determine which ear has been stimulated merely by comparing the recording from the left side with that from the right. Therefore, if one ear is to be tested alone, it is essential to mask the contralateral ear. For example, if a 100 dB stimulus is delivered to a totally deaf left ear, a response is recorded if the deafness is unilateral. The stimulus crosses over to the normal right ear and is heard at approximately 60 dB (cross-talk). As in conventional pure tone audiometry, white noise (masking noise) is applied to the contralateral ear to prevent cross-talk in such circumstances.

Unfortunately, as in conventional audiometry, the use of too loud a masking noise leads to 'over-masking' and this raises the threshold of the ear under test (Osterammel, Terkildsen and Arndal, 1970). It can be very difficult to determine the correct masking level in CERA when the hearing level of the subject is unknown. In theory, one alters the masking level in 10 dB steps until the amplitude of the response no longer alters, but in clinical practice this procedure can be very time consuming and too often judgements are made as a result of little more than a guess at the masking level.

Speech or speech sounds as stimuli. Several groups have investigated the possibility of using speech or speech sounds as stimuli for CERA. Sharrard (1973) reported that the amplitude of the response was larger when meaningful, rather than reversed meaningless words, were used. There was considerable variability in the results which were probably influenced by the extent of attention. It does not seem possible reliably to predict whether a word is understood using this method. It is likely that the onset of the sound, meaningful or meaningless, has the dominating effect on the response amplitude. Friedman *et al.* (1975) have suggested that the amplitude increase is more marked on the later components of the response (P300) and that it is closely related to increasing task demands.

Spreng (1974) used 'English-spoken' vowels, generated and adjusted to the trigger pulse by a computer, to evoke slow responses. He reported that small but significant increases in amplitudes occurred using these stimuli rather than sinusoidal tones or speech noise of equivalent loudness. Nevertheless, it appears that speech intelligibility is best determined by psycho-acoustic methods although, if an objective test could be developed, it would have a considerable impact on clinical problems such as aphasia.

Subject effects

Subject variability. There is considerable inter-subject and intra-subject variability of the slow response (Davis and Zerlin, 1966). Some of the responsible factors, such as attention and habituation, are known but there appear to be other factors which are yet to be discovered. The peak to peak amplitude usually ranges from 8–20 μV. The latencies are more consistent than the amplitudes when the same subject is tested on separate occasions. The marked variations encountered in sleep and young children are discussed separately in this chapter.

Accuracy of threshold determination. The correlation between the threshold based on the slow potential and the psycho-acoustic threshold in co-operative adults is usually within 10 dB and the scatter is not large (Beagley and Knight, 1967) (Fig. 3.4). The correlation is also close in older children (Davis, 1965b; Claus, Handrock and Arentsschild., 1975), but most workers have found CERA less reliable in young children (McCandless, 1967).

Habituation. As noted by Davis and Yoshie (1963), it is found that the slow responses are larger at the beginning than at the end of a recording session. Davis and Zerlin (1966) described the effects of habituation due to prolonged stimulation in some detail and suggested methods of reducing these effects. It helps to vary the intensity and frequency of the stimuli and to try and maintain the

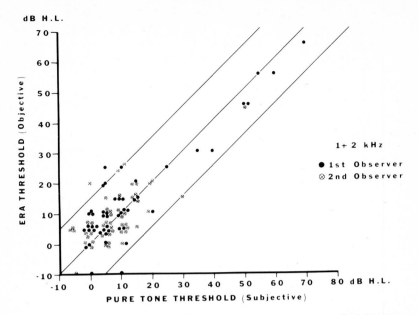

Fig. 3.4 A correlation diagram of objective and subjective thresholds on normal adults as measured by an experienced and a relatively inexperienced observer. (Beagley (1973), by permission *Minerva otorinolaryngologica*).

subject's interest in the procedure. Habituation, in these circumstances, does not affect the value of CERA and sessions lasting up to two hours can be undertaken if the subject is co-operative.

Effect of attention. Davis (1964) reported that the amplitude of the slow response increased if the subject was given a task requiring a decision but that no change was detected when the decision was simple. Mast and Watson (1968) observed that the slow potentials evoked by near threshold auditory stimuli were markedly enlarged when the subject actively listened for the stimulus. Although the earlier components of the response increase (Picton and Hillyard, 1974), the augmentation of evoked activity with attention is most pronounced as a positive wave, extending from 200–450 ms. This late positive wave is probably a composite of the P200 component evoked by the low intensity stimulus and the P300 component which is more evident when a task requiring a decision is associated with the stimulus (Freidman *et al.*, 1975). Squires, Hillyard and Lindsay (1973) have suggested that the N100 and P300 components represent different aspects of the decision process, the N100 signifying the quantity of signal information received and the P300 reflecting the confidence of the subject in performing the task correctly. A fascinating observation was made by Hillyard *et al.* (1973). They found that if a subject was asked to pay close attention to the stimulus presented to one ear but ignore any sounds presented concurrently to the opposite ear, the N100 component was substantially larger for the attended tones. This study appears to show objectively the ability of a subject to select the sound to which he listens—a necessary social asset at cocktail parties!

The test and test/retest reliability

The test reliability of CERA when used as a means of estimating the pure tone auditory threshold varies mainly with the age of the patient and the amount of patient co-operation. Most studies claim that 80–90 per cent of normally-hearing co-operative adults give CERA thresholds which are within ± 10 dB of their auditory thresholds based on psychophysical measurements (McCandless and Best, 1964; Price *et al.*, 1966; Beagley and Kellogg, 1968; *inter alia*). The most unfavourable results were those reported by Rose *et al.* (1972) who found that the agreement between CERA and psychophysical thresholds in their adult series was within 20 dB for 80 per cent of subjects but less than 70 per cent of subjects had thresholds within 10 dB. They (Rose *et al.*, 1972) also noted 11 per cent of false positive responses and, accordingly, they raised a note of caution for the interpretation of responses at near threshold levels.

The test reliability in children under the age of seven years is worse than in an adult population. Full details are given later in this chapter. Part of the problem of poor reliability in children is related to the difficulty these children have in co-operating with the lengthy test procedure whilst fully awake. This problem may also occur when testing certain groups of adults. Roeser, Price and Hnatiow (1971) found that it was often difficult to obtain CERA from adult psychiatric patients because patient movements obscured the response.

The test/retest reliability of CERA is fair. The thresholds obtained from adult co-operative patients vary little between sessions but the thresholds in young children may vary by as much as 30 dB (McCandless, 1967). The amplitude of the response varies more from session to session than the latency of the response.

Special considerations of the response in sleep

It is often necessary to test young children during sleep, as they are too active or unco-operative for the collection of the responses when they are awake. However, it is clear that the slow responses in sleep differ in many respects from those obtained from the awake subject. These differences are related to the depth of sleep and to the age of the child. In light sleep, the threshold of the response is higher than in the waking state. It is necessary, therefore, to monitor the level of sleep closely. The level of sleep can be assessed from the EEG pattern. Before interpreting the responses, it is important to consider the different EEG patterns obtained from the normal subject in the awake, waking and sleeping states.

Classification of EEG rhythms

The EEG is a record of the on-going electrical activity of the brain as obtained from electrodes placed on the scalp. If electrodes are placed directly on the exposed cortex, the electrocorticogram (ECOG) is recorded (hence the need to abbreviate electrocochleography as ECochG). The EEG is composed of a number of electrical rhythms and transient discharges which can be grouped according to their amplitude, frequency, form, periodicity and location:

Alpha (α) rhythm is greater over the occipital and parieto-occipital areas and is diminished by visual or mental activity. Its frequency is 8–13 Hz and its amplitude usually varies between 10–50 μV.

Beta (β) rhythm can be obtained from over the entire cortex. The frequency range lies mainly between 16–25 Hz and the amplitude rarely exceeds 30 μV.

Theta (θ) rhythm, not often encountered in normal alert subjects, is derived over the parietal and temporal areas. The waves have a low amplitude (less than 30 μV) and a frequency of 4–8 Hz.

Delta (Δ) rhythm is often seen during the deep stages of sleep and is most easily obtained from electrodes placed near the vertex. These waves have large amplitudes of over 100 μV and an irregular timing; the frequency range is between 0.5–3.5 Hz. Intracranial disorders, such as tumours, may generate delta rhythm in awake subjects. These large waves make CERA difficult in subjects with brain damage, etc.

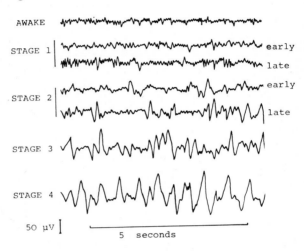

Fig. 3.5 Different EEG rhythms encountered during sleep stages.

The EEG activity during sleep

When a subject falls asleep, the EEG undergoes distinct changes which can be classified according to the depth of the sleep (Fig. 3.5):

Stage W corresponds to the waking stage. There is low voltage mixed frequency EEG activity. Some subjects exhibit continuous alpha activity whilst others may show little or none of this rhythm. Eyeblinks and EMG potentials due to tonic neck movements are common.

Stage 1 most often occurs during the transition between the waking stage and the deeper sleep stages. It usually lasts for less than ten minutes. It is characterised by low voltage, mixed frequency EEG activity of mainly 2–7 Hz but as stage 2 approaches 12–14 Hz activity may appear. Occasional sharp vertex waves are encountered. Rapid eye movements (REM) are absent although during the early stages some slow, rolling eye movements may occur.

Stage 2 is characterised by the presence of sleep spindles and often K-complexes. Sleep spindles are bursts of 12–14 Hz activity lasting over half a second. K-complexes can occur in response to sudden stimuli including auditory stimuli (Davis *et al.*, 1939). K-complexes are EEG waveforms that possess a

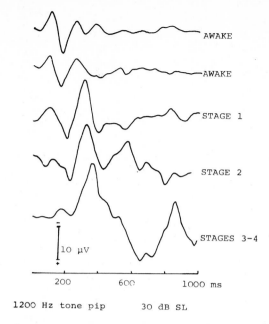

AWAKE

AWAKE

STAGE 1

STAGE 2

STAGES 3-4

10 μV

200   600   1000 ms

1200 Hz tone pip   30 dB SL

Fig. 3.6 The slow cortical responses recorded at different stages of sleep. (adapted from Osterhammel *et al*. (1973)).

sharp negative deflection followed by a positive component; each complex does not exceed half a second in duration. The high voltage activity seen in later stages does not occur.

Stage 3 is defined by an EEG in which 20–50 per cent of those waves which exceed 75 μV in amplitude are slower than 2 Hz. Sometimes sleep spindles are encountered.

Stage 4 is defined by an EEG in which more than 50 per cent of the record consists of waves slower than 2 Hz which have amplitudes of over 75 μV.

Stage REM is the stage of rapid eye movements. This stage can be related to periods of dreaming. Often distinctive sawtooth waves appear at the vertex and in the frontal regions together with the EOG potentials caused by REM.

It is not surprising that CERA under sedation can lead to difficulties in identification of 'true' responses. Davis (1973) summarised the current views regarding the use of sedation. He stated that for some young and hyperactive children sedation provided the only possible means of completing the test procedure and in these circumstances was better than no CERA at all.

A general effect is that the latency of the various components of the response increases as the depth of sleep increases. Figure 3.6 shows some typical configurations. If one considers the variability of the response encountered in young children, it is easy to recognise the problem in identifying the true responses in young sedated children. Large potentials due to REM, sleep spindles or large voltage peaks common in stage 4 sleep may swamp the averaged trace and cause fluctuations of the baseline and can be easily mistaken for true responses. Drugs, moreover, tend to elevate the threshold of the response and to increase the beta and theta EEG activity which obscures the response.

Natural sleep is reported as causing little alteration of the response characteristics (Skinner and Antinoro, 1969), but unfortunately, with the exception of young babies who may fall asleep after feeds, it is seldom possible to test a patient in these circumstances.

The ideal sedative is not yet known. Its properties would include rapid action and recovery with no after effects and it should not affect the response (Burian and Gestring, 1971). Several different agents have been evaluated (Burian, Gestring and Hruby, 1970). Rapin and Graziani (1967) found that pentobarbital sodium obscured the response in babies. Diazepam (Valium ®) was not successful in inducing sleep in 30 per cent of children (Burian and Gestring, 1971). Several groups (Stange, 1972; Karnahl and Benning, 1972; Beagley, Fateen and Gordon, 1972) favour the use of promethazine hydrochloride (Atosil ® or Phenergan ®). Beagley *et al.* (1972) recommend an intramuscular dosage of 1 mg per kg body weight. This drug appears to produce less change in the response latency and less amplitude reduction than most other agents.

In conclusion, it is probable that the choice of the sedative is less important than controlling and clearly stating the depth of the sedation induced. There is still a wide disagreement as to which stage of sleep should be recommended. Osterhammel *et al.* (1973) found the responses to be easily detected in deep sleep, whilst Salomon, Beck and Elberling, 1973, reported that the interpretation of the recordings in deep sleep was hazardous as artefacts frequently occurred which could be easily mistaken for true responses. Ritvo, Ornitz and Walter (1967) have suggested that CERA is best performed at the time of onset of sleep to reduce the number of false results.

Special considerations concerning children

CERA is certainly a reliable means of estimating the hearing levels of adults and older children, and even inexperienced workers have little difficulty in obtaining clear responses from their colleagues or other 'volunteers'. An objective audiometric test, however, is more urgently required for those young children who cannot be assessed with certainty using subjective or behavioural tests alone. Unfortunately, the estimation of threshold levels in young children is a difficult task which often lacks the objectivity sought from the procedure. The most relevant of the problems encountered are now discussed in some detail.

Maturation of the slow potential

During the first few months of life profound morphological changes occur within the CNS. This maturation is reflected to some extent by changes in the slow cortical potentials. In general, the younger the age of the subject, the smaller the amplitude of the response, and the longer and more variable the latency of the components (Engel and Young, 1969; Ferriss *et al.*, 1967).

Davis and Onishi (1969) reported their findings according to conceptual age. The vertex potential was recorded first at 23–29 weeks when N1 had a latency of 180–270 ms and P2 had a latency of 600–900 ms. After 35–37 weeks, the P2 component became most prominent with a latency of approximately 300 ms. At 40 weeks (normal birth date), the P1 and N2 components were discernable, but, at 45 weeks, the N1 became indistinct again and the P2 remained the largest component with a latency of approximately 250 ms. Further decreases in the latency of the components occur chiefly over the ensuing four months. Until the age of seven or eight years is reached, the late components of the response predominate (Beagley and Kellogg, 1968) but after this age the adult waveform is attained and it becomes much simpler to identify the response.

Weitzman, Graziani and Duhamel (1967) have suggested that the different patterns of the slow cortical responses could be grouped according to gestational age and so be used to provide an estimate of CNS maturation. Morrell (1965) suggested that the maturation of the response was partly due to the position of the auditory cortex, which shifts backwards relative to skull growth, and partly due to a predominance of activity from the medial geniculate body in early stages of maturation. It is believed that thalamo-cortical interactions do not develop fully until the infant is several months old.

Instability of the waveform

The waveform of the response in young children shows marked variability and rapid changes may occur due to sudden alteration of the psychophysical state of the subjects (McCandless and Best, 1966). Presumably subject maturation is the most significant factor since several investigators have reported greater stability of the responses from older children. Davis *et al*. (1967) reported their strong impression that patterns stabilised after the age of eight years. If severe deafness is suspected, it is often advisable to begin by using a tactile stimulus so that a template can be employed for recognising possible auditory responses. Unfortunately the situation is still complicated by the lack of repeatable responses and considerable expertise is required to judge the presence or lack of a response. Further factors contributing to the instability and difficulty in recognition of the responses are discussed in the ensuing paragraphs.

High voltage background activity

Sudden fluctuations of the background activity are difficult to suppress using averaging techniques, especially if less than 100 epochs are involved, and these fluctuations appear on the 'final' averaged trace. This type of artefact obscures the waveform of the true response and, much worse, may easily masquerade as a 'true' response in a deaf child.

Young children often have a high background of EEG activity (Davis *et al*., 1967). Appleby (1964) has suggested that the amplitude of the response decreases with increasing background EEG activity but this work was not confirmed by Davis *et al*. (1966). It is the sudden spiky potentials appearing in the EEG which most commonly obscure the response. Some children even generate a peculiar type of interference consisting of large DC shifts which appear at irregular intervals with no apparent cause. The problems are most apparent on testing children with brain damage or epilepsy who often display delta EEG rhythms. These children are usually impossible to test reliably.

Muscle activity is another source of high voltage fluctuations and it is often stated that neck movements must be prohibited during testing. It is, however, unreasonable to expect a young active child to remain immobile during test periods. Often they grow so restless that attempts to keep them still end with tantrums which curtail the test. Some children with muscle spasms or tics (including athetosis) are impossible to test. Finally, movement of the electrodes or the leads causes further background fluctuations.

Various attempts have been made to limit and reject artefacts from the recordings and most systems rely on a time delay before each response is fed to the averager, during which high amplitude artefacts can be recognised (Satterfield, 1966; Shepherd, Wever and McCarren, 1970). Today, most commercially-built equipment (Madsen ERA model 74; Medelec-Amplaid ERA equipment) includes this necessary facility but the problem remains that, if too many responses are rejected, the test period becomes so prolonged that the child grows restless.

Sedation will prevent the loss of subject co-operation and lessen muscular artefacts but it does have marked effects on the EEG which often result in raising the background noise from this source.

Subject co-operation

Young children are usually apprehensive when they are restrained so that electrodes can be attached. They often dislike the scratching of the skin surface that is necessary to lower the skin/electrode resistance. Undoubtedly, workers with several years of experience can gain the confidence of many children, but casual testers will soon become disillusioned. The problem is usually intensified by the fact that CERA is more commonly requested for those children who have failed to co-operate on behavioural testing. Few children can tolerate a session lasting more than one hour; they start to fidget and then to struggle so that eventually the electrodes are dislodged and the test has to be abandoned. Most workers restrict the test to only one or two frequencies delivered to each ear.

Accuracy of threshold estimations

If CERA is to be used to estimate the hearing level of a young child, it is essential to determine the accuracy and reliability of the method. It has been found that the threshold of the slow response compares closely with the psycho-acoustic threshold obtained by conventional audiometry in older children aged 6–13 years: the mean difference is 2.2 dB and virtually all the predictions are within 15 dB (Davis *et al.*, 1967). Unfortunately this accuracy is not achieved in younger children and the gap between psycho-acoustic thresholds and CERA threshold appears to increase with decreasing age.

Children under the age of 6 tend to have a CERA threshold that is 20–30 dB worse than that obtained by conventional techniques (Beagley, 1972). Under the age of 2, there can be difficulty in recognising the responses and most workers report that the threshold levels are poorer than those obtained by other means (McCandless, 1967). Jones *et al.* (1975) report the best results to date using CERA in late infancy; they succeeded in recording responses within 20 dB of the assumed psycho-acoustic threshold in all the children they tested. Some caution is necessary, however, since it has been found that test-retest thresholds can vary by as much as 30 dB (McCandless, 1967).

Neonates are difficult to assess using CERA. Appleby (1964) studied the CERA thresholds in 40 neonates aged between 2–10 days. He reported that 85 per cent of these infants showed a response to a stimulus of 50 dB, only 40 per cent gave responses at 40 dB, and that responses could not be reliably detected below 40 dB. Similar results were obtained from sedated children by Barnet and Goodwin (1965) and Suzuki, Tanaka and Arayama (1966).

Subject state

A simple answer to the problem of subject co-operation in young children would appear to be sedation. The effects of the different stages of sleep have already been discussed in detail in this chapter and, when these effects are added to the variability of the response in young children, it is not surprising to learn that there is a good deal of conflict in the literature concerning the ideal sedative and depth of sleep required for CERA in young children. Skinner and Antinoro (1969) found the response was clearer when obtained from the sedated child, and they attributed this finding to a reduction in the voltage of the ongoing EEG activity. Rapin and Bergman (1969) found that the response amplitude was larger when the EEG contained high voltage activity. Cohen *et al.* (1971) reported that the recognition of responses was most difficult when the EEG activity was desynchronised, as it is during the REM stage of sleep. In general it is found that although the response may have a greater amplitude in sleep, care has to be taken to control the depth of sleep and to monitor the EEG activity to prevent sudden large fluctuations from being included into the averaged trace and mistakenly interpreted as a true response. The technique of CERA in sedated children and the recognition of the responses requires considerable skill and, even when this is acquired, the reliability of CERA in indicating the psycho-acoustic threshold is poor.

Instrumentation

The instrumentation required for CERA has been described in Chapter 2, so it is only necessary to mention the details which are specific.

The test environment

Subjects should be tested in a comfortable relaxed position. Adults and older children are seated in a chair with a pillow placed under the neck to reduce neck movements which may result in myogenic potentials. Infants and sedated subjects are usually tested whilst lying on a coach under close supervision. The room should ideally be sound proofed but it is possible to get worthwhile results providing any quiet environment is available.

Stimulus generation

Stimulus envelope.   Pure tone stimuli are used. The most commonly recommended stimulus envelope has a rise and decay time of 25–30 ms and a plateau of 25–50 ms. The largest response amplitudes are obtained using the lower audiometric frequencies (0.25–2 kHz).

Stimulus repetition rate.   Due to the slow recovery time of the slow response, it is not possible to use fast repetition rates. The rate chosen is therefore a compromise between the reduction in the response amplitude caused by fast stimulus rates and the clinical need to limit the period of testing. A rate of one stimulus every one or two seconds is commonly recommended.

Number of stimulus presentations.   Often, between 30 and 70 stimuli must be presented before a clear averaged response can be detected, the larger number being necessary when using stimuli at intensites close to the psycho-acoustic threshold. It takes between half a minute to two minutes to collect the necessary number of responses.

Stimulus transducer.   Adults and older children can be tested using a pair of earphones so that monaural information can be obtained. Masking of the non-test ear is required at high intensities. It is possible to use a bone conductor to obtain responses but care has to be taken not to record a false bone conduction threshold in a deaf subject due to a tactile rather than an auditory input. Young children may be best tested using a free-field loudspeaker if they show signs of not tolerating the earphones.

Stimulus calibration.   The calibration of the tone bursts used for CERA is a simple matter compared with that of calibrating clicks and several methods may be used. Most clinicians prefer a biological calibration corresponding to ISO recommendations, as the results of CERA can then be compared directly with pure tone audiometry (PTA). A simple technique is to match the amplitude of the stimulus to that of the clinic audiometer using a peak to peak comparison on an oscilloscope, but this method does depend on the clinic audiometer being, itself, accurately calibrated, and does not account for the difference in temporal integration between the short CERA stimuli and the longer PTA stimuli.

Masking (random) noise.   Masking facilities must be available if monaural information is sought when the thresholds of the two ears vary by more than 40 dB. Narrow band masking noise based on the test frequency is usually delivered to the non-test ear to prevent cross-talk.

The recording equipment

Electrodes.   Surface electrodes are required and any high quality EEG electrodes can be used. Commonly silver/silver chloride dome electrodes are employed. Kado and Adey (1968) have suggested that tin/tin chloride electrodes are better as they reduce the skin/electrode impedance, but their suggestion has not been commercialised. The active electrode can be placed anywhere within 6–8 cm of the vertex (Cody and Klass, 1968) but most workers use a site 1 cm in front of the vertex in the midline. The reference electrode may be placed on the mastoid or earlobe (Goff *et al.*, 1969) and it may be on either side of the head. The earth electrode is usually placed on the nasion. The electrode/skin impedance should be less than 5 kΩ.

Amplifiers.   Low noise biological amplifiers are essential. The total gain necessary is 10^5 approximately using Medelec MkII amplifiers. Often a pre-amplifier with a fixed gain is placed close to the patient and the final gain adjustment is made on an amplifier housed with the averager. Reneau and Mast

(1968) and other workers have used a biotelemetry transmitter and receiver placed between the pre-amplifier and main amplifier when testing retarded subjects to prevent them becoming distracted by the connecting wires.

Filter settings.   The low pass filter should be set at approximately 13.6 Hz which is low enough to prevent much interference from mains electricity sources. The high pass filter is usually set at 1.6 Hz which is just high enough to avoid troublesome DC disturbances. Unfortunately these filter settings enhance the EEG background activity but this is inevitable when one considers the source of the response.

Averager.   There are many computers and purpose-built averagers than can be used for CERA. The analysis period should be 1000 ms with a delay of 250 ms displayed before the stimulus onset so that the background activity can be assessed (Rose and Rittmanic, 1968). It is possible to use a shorter analysis period when testing co-operative adult subjects.

Monitor oscilloscope.   A monitor oscilloscope on which the on-going EEG rhythm is displayed is essential; with it, it is then possible to detect changes in the EEG activity which may contaminate the averaged recording. If subjects are sedated, it is important that the stage of sleep is monitored throughout the test session and many workers advocate that a permanent recording of these details should be available.

It is helpful if the response is displayed during the actual process of averaging as it takes little practice to detect the sudden changes in the baseline caused by an artefact which can otherwise mistakenly be interpreted as a response.

Artefact rejection facilities.   Sudden voltages caused by movements or from other sources can be limited or excluded from the averager if artefact rejection facilities are available. These facilities can help identification considerably when young children are being tested, although the criteria for accepting a response must not be so stringent as to prolong the test session unduly.

Permanent recording of results.   Permanent records are useful as they can be used for further analysis after the test session. The analysis period, polarity, amplitude calibration and any stimulus delay should always be noted together with all other important subject and test details.

Testing procedures

Adults are usually easy to test, but young children can be very difficult.

Adults are usually co-operative and are tested whilst sitting comfortably in a chair with the neck relaxed against a pillow. They are asked not to to move during the averaging period of each response or trial. Because a notable feature of the slow potential is the variability of its amplitude, occasionally subjects are encountered with tiny responses which can make interpretation very difficult. It may help in these circumstances to ask the subject to perform a mental task such as reading or arithmetic. It is important to realise that masking of the contralateral ear is as necessary as with conventional audiometry whenever monaural information is sought.

Children under the age of six are often difficult to test. As already mentioned the long duration of the CERA procedure is taxing for the young child and gives great opportunity for the response to be affected by random background electrical events such as may be evoked by movements. A great deal of skill is needed in the management of these young children and this is not acquired except by experience. Some workers are able to gain the co-operation of the majority of seemingly unruly children, but the worker beginning in this field must be prepared for the frustration of failure.

Interpretaion of threshold

The threshold of the potential in CERA is detected by first commencing testing using a stimulus intensity which is, one hopes, well above the audible threshold. The stimulus intensity is then reduced from trial to trial in 20 dB steps until the threshold is crossed as shown by a clearly negative trial, i.e. the absence of a visible slow potential (Fig. 3.7). The stimulus intensity may be altered in smaller steps of 5–10 dB at intensities close to threshold if a more accurate level is sought. Clinically, thresholds are often determined at 500 Hz, 1000 Hz and

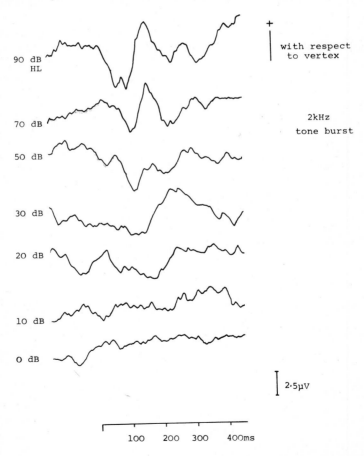

Fig. 3.7 An example of using the slow cortical response to detect threshold.

2000 Hz as this gives a good indication of the hearing in the important speech range. The thresholds to other frequencies can be determined, but this can prolong the procedure to such an extent that it becomes impracticable. The main problem with the exact interpretation of the threshold intensity level is that the amplitude of the slow potential is minute close to threshold and easily obscured by background electrical events.

When a deaf child is tested it may be necessary to obtain a tactile response as a preliminary before a confident conclusion concerning the absence of an auditory response can be reached. Most workers suggest that the averaged response should be carefully monitored during 'building' on the screen of the oscilloscope so that random fluctuations can be recognised and discounted. Kawamura *et al.* (1972) suggest that the averaged response should be displayed after 50, 100, 150 and 200 stimuli and that only if the response grows consistently should it be accepted. Unfortunately such a prolonged procedure is rarely clinically feasible. The author uses the technique which is available on the Medelec-Amplaid equipment of directing the response to alternate stimuli to different stores of the averager (A and B). The waveform of the response in each store is compared with the other for consistency before adding them together for the final result.

It is possible that a computer could be programmed to identify true evoked potentials more efficiently than is possible subjectively (Salomon, 1975). This method would then provide a truly objective form of audiometry. At present no definite programme is available and it is unlikely that such a method will be cost effective for the average clinic, especially as there are alternative forms of ERA available.

The clinical use of CERA

CERA may be used as a means of estimating the auditory acuity and direct comparison can be made with the results of conventional pure tone audiometry. Attempts have also been made to develop CERA as a neuro-otological tool but scant success has been met in this field.

As a means of estimating auditory acuity
CERA is a useful audiometric technique in adults and older children and it is indicated in the following cases:

1. Confused or uncomprehending subjects who are unable to follow the instructions for conventional audiometry.
2. Unreliable subjects who give varying subjective thresholds. CERA will indicate the true threshold.
3. Unduly passive subjects who will not respond reliably during audiometric testing. CERA is very easy with such a person.
4. Suspected 'hysterical' or 'non-organic' hearing loss.
5. In medico-legal cases to confirm the subjective audiometric results and to detect any malingering. These latter indications, (4 and 5 are arguably the clearest for the clinical use of CERA in present clinical practice.)

There are many reports which show an excellent correlation between CERA and the results obtained by conventional pure tone audiometric techniques and these have been mentioned earlier in this chapter. Rose *et al*. (1972) found that 70 per cent of their CERA estimates were within 10 dB of the subjective threshold but they did express concern that 11 per cent of the non-stimulus trials were reported as giving a (false) positive response.

In children under the age of six, many difficulties are encountered on using CERA to estimate the auditory acuity and these have already been mentioned. At present most workers believe that the following conditions are contraindications to the use of CERA in children:

1. Epilepsy.
2. Muscle tics or spasms, e.g. athetosis.

These two conditions are usually associated with numerous electrical artefacts which make interpretation of the responses hazardous.

3. Some forms of brain damage associated with large amplitude slow EEG waves which tend to be easily confused with the response.

4. At present the need for *sedation* is probably a contraindication. Most workers prefer the use of another form of ERA (ECochG, BER or the middle latency responses).

As a means of neuro-otological diagnosis

The variability of the slow potential makes the interpretation of changes due to specific pathological conditions difficult in the individual case but some conclusions have been reached after comparing the results obtained from groups of subjects with the same disorder and a group of normal subjects.

Conductive hearing losses. Slow vertex potentials evoked by use of a vibrator placed on the mastoid area can be recorded. It is hoped that a 'bone conduction' (BC) threshold can be obtained which is directly comparable to the subjective pure tone bone conduction threshold. Cody, Griffing and Taylor (1968) examined CERA bone conduction thresholds in 28 normal ears at frequencies of 500, 1000 and 2000 Hz and reported that the thresholds obtained were within 15 dB of the subjective BC threshold in 95 per cent of the cases. In patients with a severe sensorineural hearing loss, it is possible that the response may be evoked by a tactile rather than by an auditory pathway (Townsend and Cody, 1970). Some caution is therefore necessary even when masking has been applied correctly.

Cochlear disorders. Pathological conditions which affect the cochlea are often characterised by the phenomenon of recruitment (Dix, Hallpike and Hood, 1948), in which a relatively small increase in the sound intensity results in a larger increase in the psycho-acoustic sensation of loudness.

Clayton and Rose (1970) found no differences between the amplitude and latency functions of CERA responses to the same loud stimulus when it was presented to normally hearing ears or to ears with suspected cochlear hearing losses. Knight and Beagley (1968) have shown that the amplitude/intensity functions of the slow potential rise abnormally steeply in recruiting types of hearing loss and so resemble the subjective Fowler's alternate binaural loudness balance test (Fig. 3.8). Uziel (1975) mentioned that the enlargment of the slow response was most marked in recruiting ears within 20 dB of the response threshold. These are findings based on the averaged results from groups of subjects. Unfortunately, the variability of the response makes diagnosis difficult in the individual case but it can be said with reasonable confidence that, if the evoked response is traced down towards its threshold in a partially hearing subject and there is a sudden 'collapse' of amplitude as the threshold is approached, recruitment is indeed present.

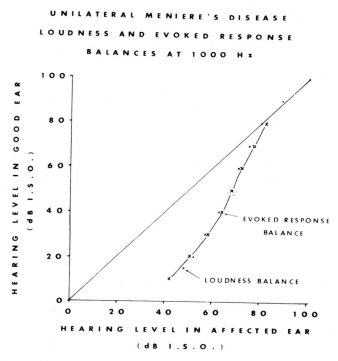

Fig. 3.8 A comparison of equal loudness balance (Fowler's test) and equal CERA amplitude balance in a subject with a recruiting hearing loss (Knight, J.J. & Beagley, H.A. (1968), by permission *Audiology*).

Ménière's disorder.   A syndrome involving a triad of symptoms: hearing loss, tinnitus and vertigo, was first described by Ménière (1861). Histological studies have associated this syndrome in some instances with endolymphatic hydrops. When the aetiology of the condition is unknown (idiopathic), the term Ménière's disorder is often applied.

It has been reported that groups of patients with Ménière's disorder have, on average, shorter response latencies than groups of normally hearing subjects (Townsend and Cody, 1970; Shimizu, 1968). This finding, however, cannot be applied easily to individual cases and in any case is not pathognomonic of Ménière's disorder as it has been noted in a wide variety of sensorineural conditions. Best and Tabor (1968) examined the recovery function of the P2 (P200) component using paired stimuli at varying interstimulus intervals (ISI).

They reported that normal subjects and patients with conductive hearing losses showed a dip in the recovery function at 800 ms ISI; patients with cochlear disorders gave a dip at 400 ms ISI and patients with retrocochlear lesions had a dip at 200 ms ISI. Townsend and Cody (1970) repeated this work but could not confirm the findings; in particular, they noted that many patients with Ménière's disorder gave a dip in their recovery functions at 200 ms ISI.

VIII nerve disorders. Shimizu (1968) after testing four patients suggested that the latency of the response was increased and its amplitude diminished when retrocochlear pathology was present. Townsend and Cody (1970) could only confirm this finding in one of their six cases.

Central disorders. It is still hoped that alterations in the functions of the slow potential may indicate disorders of the cerebrum but no clear results have yet been described which can help the clinician in his evaluation of the individual case. Beagley (1974) found no obvious difference on comparing the responses from a group of aphasic children with those of a group of normally hearing children.

Morrison, Gibson and Beagley (1976) report a use of CERA together with electrocochleography in localising a lesion. A patient with a large centrally-placed tumour and subjective hearing loss gave an apparently normal transtympanic electrocochleogram. CERA was useful in that it confirmed the subjective threshold and so excluded the possibility of a non-organic hearing loss and placed the lesion between the eighth nerve and the auditory cortex.

Final remarks

The slow cortical response has many limitations as a clinical test. The variability of the response, especially its amplitude, latency and waveform, and the difficulties in identifying true responses when the spurious background electrical activity is high have led to disillusionment. The worker with CERA encounters problems especially in the very group of unco-operative young children in which the need for accurate auditory assessment is most urgent, and the slow potential is not sufficiently uniform to allow its use as a neuro-otological tool in individual subjects. Despite these difficulties, it must be remembered that CERA provides an accurate prediction of the pure tone audiogram in adults and older children, so its real value probably lies at present with the objective assessment of possible non-organic hearing loss and with medico-legal compensation cases. In the future, perhaps, the problems curtailing its use in the sedated young child will be solved and its use in neuro-otological diagnosis will be established. CERA would then become a much more valuable technique and would regain favour amongst clinical workers.

4. Electrocochleography (E Coch G)

Electrocochleography (ECochG) is a method of recording of the electrical activity of the cochlea and first order, eighth nerve fibres in response to acoustic stimulation. The electrical responses from higher levels of the auditory tract have been deliberately excluded from this definition.

ECochG is proving to be one of the most valuable ERA techniques currently available to the clinician and provides an accurate, easily identifiable measure of the threshold of cochlear function which may be used confidently to estimate hearing acuity. The potentials recorded are not affected by sedation and no masking of the contralateral ear is necessary. These features combine to form a very robust tool for the paedo-audiologist. It is possible to test objectively the cochlear function of *any child*, even in the presence of multiple handicaps, providing that child is able to undergo a general anaesthetic.

The clinical use of ECochG is not restricted to measurement of threshold. Detailed analyses of ECochG responses show consistent variations in several types of hearing impairment. It is hoped that ECochG will prove useful for diagnostic purposes, and that it will serve the otologist in a few years hence in the same manner as electrocardiography (ECG) serves the cardiologist of today. ECochG may also be used to monitor the electrophysiological changes which occur within the cochlea after some event such as the infusion of a drug. This application has been used widely in animal studies, but it is only recently that the ECochG has been used to monitor effects on the human cochlea (Ramsden, Wilson and Gibson, 1977).

The history of the subject has been mentioned in some detail in Chapter One. Briefly, the cochlear microphonic (CM) was described first by Wever and Bray (1930), and Saul and Davis (1932) were the first to distinguish the action potential (AP). Many years later, the summating potential (SP) was independently described by Davis, Fernãndez and McAuliffe (1950) and by Békésy (1950). Attempts to measure these potentials in man (Lempert *et al.*, 1950) met with little success until the introduction of the averaging computer. In 1967, several laboratories (Portmann, Le Bert and Aran, 1967; Yoshie, Ohashi and Suzuki, 1967; Sohmer and Feinmesser, 1967; Spreng and Keidel, 1967) simultaneously published reports of obtaining the ECochG in man with minimal surgical intervention. Within the last few years, there has been an enormous expansion of research into the field and rapid strides are being made in the understanding and clinical application of the subject.

The anatomy and physiology of the cochlea

The anatomy

The bony cochlea lies within the petrous temporal bone. It resembles the shape of a snail's shell and, in man, it coils for 2¾ turns for a distance of approximately 35 mm. Its basal turn forms the promontory part of the medial surface of the middle ear, and its apex is directed towards the internal acoustic meatus. The coil is formed around a central bony axis known as the modiolus, which is thick at the base but narrows towards the apex.

An osseous spiral lamina projects from the modiolus into the cochlea resembling the thread of a screw. The modiolus is traversed by numerous minute canals and by a larger canal which runs lengthwise in the centre. The spiral lamina also contains small canals which communicate with those in the modiolus. One canal, named the spiral canal of the modiolus, winds spirally around the modiolus in the attached margin of the spiral lamina and contains the spiral ganglion, a long spiralling structure.

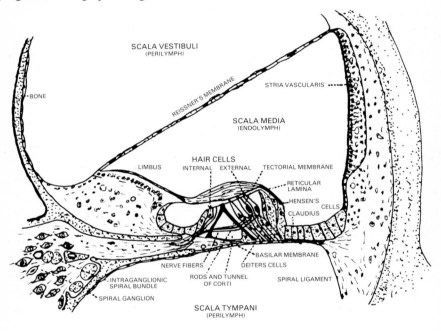

Fig. 4.1 Cross-sectional drawing of the canal at the second turn of a guinea pig's cochlea (Adapted from Davis *et al*. (1953)).

The osseous cochlea contains perilymph and encloses the membraneous cochlea which contains endolymph. The membranous cochlea is in continuity, via the ductus reuniens, with the saccule, utricle and semicircular canals. It is bounded by the osseous spiral lamina, Reissner's membrane, the stria vascularis and the basilar membrane (Fig. 4.1). The membranous cochlea does not extend along the entire length of the osseous cochlea in mammals, as it ends just before the apex and here, at the helicotrema, the perilymph of the scala vestibuli and the scala tympani are in continuity.

Set upon the basilar membrane is the organ of Corti, the sense organ of hearing, which extends the whole length of the membranous cochlea. There are three main structures; the sensory hair bearing cells which sit astride the pillars of the tunnel of Corti, supporting cells, and the overlying gelatinous tectorial membrane. In man, the sensory cells are arranged as a single row of inner hair cells and three rows of outer hair cells, and there are approximately 25 000 hair cells in each organ of Corti (Chow, 1951). Minute hairs, 4 μ long and 0.1 μ thick, project from the upper surface of the outer hair cells and are embedded into the tectorial membrane whilst the hairs of the inner hair cells lie free. The space within the pillars of the tunnel of Corti contains cortilymph (Engström, 1960) which resembles perilymph both in composition and in many other respects. Von Ilberg (1968) has performed studies which show that the corticolymph communicates freely with the perilymph via minute openings in the osseous spiral lamina.

The inner hair cells are bulbous in shape and the hairs are arranged in two rows in the shape of a double V with their apices directed away from the modiolus forming a continuous chain from one hair cell to the next: there are 35–40 hairs on each inner hair cell. The outer hair cells are columnar in shape and the hairs are arranged in three rows like a wide triple W: there are approximately 115 hairs on each outer hair cell. The kinocilium of the vestibular sensory cell is represented in the hair cell by a simple basal body (Ades, Engström and Hawkins, 1962) which is difficult to identify with certainty.

The nervous connections of the organ of Corti

There are two types of nerve endings in functional contact with the hair cells (Engström, 1958; Smith and Sjöstrand, 1961). Type I is small and sparsely granulated and associated with afferent fibres carrying the neural messages to the brain, whilst type II is larger and more densely granulated and associated with

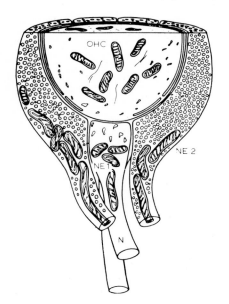

Fig. 4.2 The nerve terminals associated with an outer hair cell. NE1—afferent terminal; NE2—efferent nerve terminal (Engström *et al.* (1965), by permission Academic Press).

efferent fibres (Fig. 4.2) (Engström and Fernàndez, 1961). These efferent fibres are from the olivo-cochlear bundle and pass initially along the vestibular nerve before reaching the cochlear nerve by means of the anastomosis of Oört. The presence of the granules suggests that they may release a chemical, probably acetyl choline which alters the hair cell membrane permeability allowing the escape of potassium ions into the perilymph.

The fibre distribution within the cochlea may be classified simply into three groups, afferent, efferent and autonomic components:

1. Afferent fibres
a. The inner radial bundles—these provide afferent connections for the inner hair cells; each hair cell is related to a small number of fibres. Spoendlin (1972) found that 95 per cent of the total number of afferent fibres are distributed in this group, about 20 fibres to each inner hair cell.

b. The outer spiral fibres—the remaining 5 per cent of the afferent nerves leaving the cochlea come from the outer hair cells. These fibres originate from as many as 10 outer hair cells spread over as much as one third of a turn of the cochlea and cross the tunnel of Corti as basilar fibres. Each outer hair cell contacts the terminals of several different outer spiral fibres.

2. The efferent fibres in contrast distribute predominantly radially as tunnel radial fibres to the outer hair cells, especially those of the first row (Spoendlin, 1976). Nearly all the efferent supply to the outer hair cells originates from the contralateral brainstem, whilst the supply to the inner hair cells is derived mainly from the homolateral side of the brainstem.

3. The third group of cochlear innervation components consists of autonomic fibres originating from the superior cervical ganglion. The functional significance of these fibres is not yet known.

Physiology
There are two classic theories of pitch perception:

1. Helmholtz's 'place' theory was a revival of a theory begun over 300 years ago. Bauhin (1605) was perhaps the first to suggest that there was selective resonance in various cavities within the ear. Du Verney (1683) regarded the bony spiral lamina as the selective structure, since the manner of the distribution of the cochlear nerve to this structure was already known. Over the next hundred years, the membranous cochlear partition was recognised as the vibrating structure with the high tones perceived at the base and low tones at the apex (Cotugno, 1761). Helmholtz (1859, 1863) used Fourier's theorem, which had just been formulated, to explain how a periodic complex sound wave could be presented as a number of single tones. He suggested that there was one resonator for each tone in the cochlea and that each was connected to the brain by its own individual nerve. There are two main objections to this theory; firstly, there are insufficient fibres in the cochlear nerve to account for every single frequency, and secondly, it is known that a considerable length of basilar membrane is set into vibration by any one pure tone.

2. Rutherford's 'telephone' (1886) theory proposed that the frequency of the

sound was relayed to the brain by the corresponding number of neural impulses per second. This theory was shown to have limitations when it was found that a nerve fibre cannot carry more than 500–600 neural impulses per second. Wever (1949) extended the 'telephone' theory by proposing the 'volley' theory in which the frequency information is carried by a group of fibres, each firing rhythmically at a fraction of the speed of the frequency so that the stimulus frequency is represented in the combined pattern. There are objections to this theory especially when applied to frequencies over 3 000 Hz since the delay at synapses does not occur sufficiently regularly to allow the combined effect to be recognisable (Whitfield, 1967). In their general sense, Wever's theories are still acceptable today but there is now much more factual knowledge especially regarding the frequency selectivity of the ear and temporal coding.

Frequency selectivity may be explained as the ability of a system to resolve or separate out the individual components of a complex signal. In radio or television, this task may be accomplished by a bank of overlapping filters. Each filter rejects all frequencies higher or lower than the preset range so that only a narrow band of frequencies passes. In this manner, the individual components of a complex signal can be separated for analysis. It is suggested that the auditory system functions in a similar manner.

Psychophysical measurements known as 'critical bands' have been used to find the effective bandwidth of the auditory system. It appears that man possesses the equivalent of a bank of overlapping filters within his auditory system with critical bands ranging from 200 Hz at 1 kHz to 2 kHz at 10 kHz.

The question is: 'How and where does the auditory system achieve this fine tuning?'. The mechanical tuning of the basilar membrane has been measured by Békésy (1944) in various animals using an optical method and the results show that it is poorly tuned. Similar results have been reported using different methods: the Mössbauer technique (Johnstone and Boyle, 1967), the speckle pattern of a laser beam (Kohllöffel, 1972) and a capacative probe technique (Wilson and Johnstone, 1975). There is no doubt that the basilar membrane does not act as the sharply tuned structure required by psychophysics, nor as the resonator system originally proposed by Helmholtz (1857), but as a heavily damped, broadly tuned structure.

When Tasaki (1954) first made recordings of single fibre activity within the eighth nerve, he reported that the neural activity was broadly tuned like the basilar membrane. This led to the belief that the information leaving the ear was broadly tuned and that this information was sharpened up in some way at higher levels of the auditory system.

The more recent recordings of single nerve activity have shown the findings of Tasaki (1954) to be largely erroneous (Katsuki *et al.*, 1958; Kiang *et al.*, 1965; De Boer, 1969; Evans, Rosenberg and Wilson, 1970). These workers have found that the tuning of the single cochlear nerve fibres at near threshold levels is sufficiently fine to meet the psychophysical requirements (Fig. 4.3). There must therefore be a second filter mechanism within the cochlea which accounts for the difference between the tuning of the basilar membrane and the tuning of the afferent nerve activity (Evans and Wilson, 1973). The presence of this second filter is of great

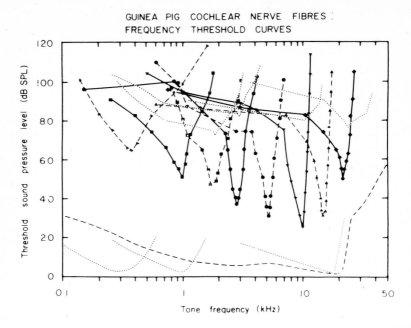

Fig. 4.3 Single nerve fibre tuning curves. Upper complete lines--normal fibres. Upper dotted lines—fibres rendered anoxic. Lower incomplete lines—basilar membrane tuning (Evans, E.F. (1975a), by permission *Academic Press*).

importance to ECochG. It also provides the most satisfactory explanation of the presence of recruitment in such conditions as Ménière's disorder. The matter is discussed further on page 77.

At higher intensity levels, the neural tuning of the cochlea is broad and cannot match the psychophysical tuning. It seems probable that there is some further tuning mechanism within the CNS for these high intensities. It may be that the efferent system acts by lateral inhibition to narrow the shoulders of the tuning curves and there is some recent evidence that this may occur within the nuclei of the brainstem.

Temporal (time) coding involves the ability of the ear to detect time varying events. A useful aid is the post-stimulus-time (PST) histogram which shows the number of neural fibres activated at each moment after the stimulus. Studies of the PST histogram reveal that a single fibre unit response is instantaneously related to the upward (towards the scala vestibuli) movement of the basilar membrane caused by the rarefaction phase of a stimulus (when the stapes footplate is moving outwards).

If one plots the probability of neural discharge during a stimulus cycle of a sinusoidal tone, it is obvious that discharges occur only during the rarefaction phases and so the PST histogram has been named under these circumstances, the period or cycle histogram. The time delays between each neural discharge are known as the interval histogram. It seems likely that the auditory system can analyse this periodicity of neural firing to obtain further information, which may be especially useful in the low frequency domains.

The mechanical vibration of the basilar membrane

The basic assumption has been made (Békésy, 1947) that the cochlear fluids vibrate instantaneously from window to window without significant compression or rarefaction of its constituent molecules. Wever and Lawrence (1954) showed by drilling various observation holes in the cochlear wall, that the behaviour of the inner ear was quite unaffected by the point at which the vibrations were applied to the cochlear fluids. The mechanical drive of the basilar membrane is not provided directly by movements of the stapes but comes from the pressure changes in the fluids of the cochlea. The mode of fluid vibrations has now been accepted as being in accordance with Békésy's (1947) finding of a travelling wave. This wave begins from the basal end of the basilar membrane and travels towards the apex (regardless of the site of the initiating vibration). At very low frequencies, the whole basilar membrane vibrates but as the driving frequency is increased, so the rate of change of phase with distance increases and a wavetrain of several cycles develops. The wave rises slowly on the basal side and falls abruptly on the apical side, rather like a wave from the sea approaching the beach. The point at which the wave 'breaks' moves progressively apically along the basilar membrane as the frequency is lowered (Fig. 4.4), the force that the wave exerts on the basilar membrane being dependent both on the amplitude and the phase angle of the wave.

The velocity of sound waves in the cochlear fluids is approximately 1 500 metres/second, so the time of transmission along the whole length of the cochlea in man is about 30 microseconds. Thus, regardless of the site of the driving vibration, the pressure is applied virtually simultaneously along the whole length of the basilar membrane. The travelling wave has a much slower velocity. Zerlin (1969) has estimated the travelling wave velocity from psycho-acoustically obtained data and Eggermont and Odenthal (1974) produced similar data based on their findings using electrocochleography. Although the actual mean velocity of the travelling wave varies with frequency, in general its velocity is 30 metres per second in the basal turn and 1 metre per second near the apex. In a guinea pig the wave takes approximately 2 milliseconds to travel the 18mm from the oval window to the apex (Whitfield, 1967); in man, the cochlea measures some 35mm, so one may expect the travelling wave to take approximately 4 milliseconds to

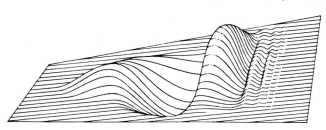

Fig. 4.4 A diagrammatical representation of the travelling wave. (After Tonndorf, J. (1962), by permission *Journal of the Acoustical Society of America*).

cover the distance from oval window to apex. These findings are of particular relevance to electrocochleography.

The cochlear transducer mechanism

In some manner, as yet incompletely understood, the mechanical vibrations of the basilar membrane effect a discharge of neural impulses in the cochlear nerve. The travelling wave distorts the basilar membrane on which the hair cells lie. The hairs of the outer hair cells are embedded in the tectorial membrane which, being unattached at one end, is not distorted and the hairs are bent due to the shearing action between the basilar membrane and the tectorial membrane (Fig. 4.5). The hairs of the inner hair cells are displaced by movement of the cochlear fluids. The bending of the hairs is known to be related to the earliest of electrical potentials observed in the cochlea, the cochlear microphonic.

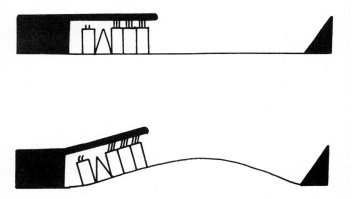

Fig. 4.5 A model of the bending of cilia following basilar membrane movement.

The cochlear microphonic

A crystal microphone transduces acoustic waveforms into their electronic waveforms with an accuracy which is appropriate to the quality of the device. In a similar manner it appears that the hair cells of the cochlea change the mechanical vibrations of the basilar membrane into their electrical waveforms. Both the microphonic recorded from an individual hair cell (not yet accomplished in practice) and the microphonic recorded from the region of the round window may be termed 'cochlear microphonic'. There are, nevertheless several differences between the two types of cochlear microphonic, since the round window recording represents the sum of the microphonic from many individual hair cells which are driven, especially at higher frequencies, by different phases of the travelling wave (Whitfield and Ross, 1965). This book refers specifically to the 'summed' microphonic obtained from an electrode sited at a distance from the hair cells as the 'cochlear microphonic (CM)'.

It is generally accepted that the source of the CM is the hair cells. If a microelectrode is advanced from the scala tympani through the basilar membrane, the CM remains substantially unchanged until the tip of the electrode penetrates the cuticular plate covering the upper surface of the hair cell, at which point an abrupt 180 degree phase change takes place in the recording (Tasaki, Davis and Eldredge., 1954). This and other evidence has strongly suggested that the site of the hair cell microphonic is close to the hair bearing surface of the cell. The only conflicting evidence is that of Lawrence, Nuttall and McCabe (1974) who describe the electrical changes as occurring on the surface of the tectorial membrane.

A substance, such as a quartz crystal, may generate electricity (the piezo-electric effect) when a mechanical force distorts its shape. Histologically, there are longitudinal chains of poly-saccharides within the hair cell and it has been suggested that movement of the hairs distorts these chains and produces the microphonic by. a piezo-electric phenomenon. Unfortunately, the situation cannot be quite so simple. Békésy (1947) has determined the amplitude of the vibration of the basilar membrane and found it to be in the order of 10^{-4} cm at 34 dB SPL. Assuming the system to be linear, the amplitude of vibration at the psychophysical threshold is 2×10^{-11} (1/500th of the diameter of a hydrogen atom), which is below the thermal noise of the system (Békésy and Rosenblith, 1951). The amplitude of vibration is too small to account for the microphonic purely on the basis of a piezo-electric mechanism. A further experiment performed by Békésy (1950) argues against the piezo-electric mechanism acting alone. He displaced the basilar membrane using a needle and found the potential difference caused by the displacement remained indefinitely. The hair cell microphonic was related to the degree of displacement but not the amount of work employed. This surely means that the mechanical movement of the hairs modulates some other source of energy and does not itself provide the energy. The source of the extrinsic energy may be related to the resting or steady state electrical potentials within the cochlea.

There are certain properties of the CM which must be clearly understood before one attempts to interpret the recordings obtained by electrocochleography:

1. Individual hair cells are not frequency specific. Their specificity is merely due to their position on the basilar membrane. The hair cells in the basal coil of the cochlea not only generate CM to high frequency stimulation but also to lower frequency stimuli passing up to the more apical regions.

2. The amplitude of the 'summed' CM is a resultant of the CM from many individual hair cells which are generating CM at different electrical phases. The lower the frequency of stimulation, the more hair cells will produce microphonics in the same phase, and the larger the 'summed' CM will be.

3. Dallos (1973) has suggested that the outer hair cells provide the majority of the CM recorded at the round window and the inner hair cells do not contribute to any meaningful extent.

4. The amplitude of the CM is attenuated in proportion to the distance of the recording electrode from the generator site. Békésy (1951) has suggested this attenuation is approximately 6 dB/mm in the cat and Tasaki, Davis and Legouix (1952) offered a figure of 7 dB/mm. In man, the figure is probably about 3 dB/mm within the basal turn. This attenuation is important when considering

recordings from the round window; it is probably chiefly a result of the phase dependency of each of the individual hair cell microphonics.

It must be remembered, therefore, that CM recordings in ECochG generally only relate to a limited area of basilar membrane close to the round window (Tasaki *et al.*, 1952; Simmons and Beatty, 1962), so no conclusions can be drawn from these recordings about the function of hair cells outside the basal turn. It is occasionally possible, however, to record CM activity from higher along the cochlear partition—the so-called 'remote CM'. This occurs when all the hair cells in the basal part of the cochlea have been destroyed. The CM from the nearest surviving group of hair cells is recorded as there is no attenuation of their potential by CM arising in the basal region. It is also possible in certain cases of localised hair cell loss within the basal region to record an abnormally large CM response as two adjacent surviving hair cell groups may produce CM which is essentially 'in phase'.

The summating potential

A second cochlear receptor potential has been noted in addition to the CM; this is characterised by a DC shift in the baseline of the response, generally in a negative direction, and occurs for the duration of the stimulus. Davis and his co-workers (1950) have named this response 'the summating potential'.

The summating potential (SP) is normally only present at high stimulus intensities, so it was initially postulated that its origin lay within the inner hair cells. This theory was discounted when it was shown that the avian cochlea which has no inner hair cells yielded a SP (Stopp and Whitfield, 1964). The most recent explanation is that the SP is a multi-component response which arises from various non-linear mechanisms within the cochlea. These non-linearities are enhanced at high stimulus intensities.

It seems very likely that the major component of the SP results from a non-linear vibration of the basilar membrane (Whitfield and Ross, 1965). This non-linearity leads to CM being generated disproportionately in one direction. At high intensities, the SP may exceed the CM in amplitude; this may be explained if one remembers that the CM represents the sum of individual hair cell micro-phonics over a limited area of basilar membrane. The microphonic at each hair cell is in a slightly different phase to its neighbour, and consequently does not add algebraically but as a vector quantity. The SP, however, is not phase sensitive and its amplitude is directly proportional to the amount of basilar membrane displacement so it does add algebraically. The largest CM amplitude is recorded at the point closest to the maximum hair cell displacement, whereas the SP is maximum at a more distant point where the summed effect from a large area of basilar membrane may be recorded (Davis *et al.*, 1950).

The electrical sign of the SP has led to confusion in the past as it depends entirely on the site of the recording electrodes. Most experimental work has been performed with intracochlear electrodes placed within the scala media (Davis *et al.*, 1950; Tasaki, Davis and Eldredge, 1954; Konishi and Yasuno, 1963). Kupperman (1966) used a scala tympani electrode which was referred to an electrode placed on the neck muscles and this resulted in his SP bearing the opposite electrical sign to the one described by the former workers.

Dallos, Schoeny and Cheatham (1972) have published an excellent and authoritative account of the SP. They placed their electrodes simultaneously within the scala tympani and scala vestibuli and analysed the DC potential difference across the cochlear partition (DIF SP) and the common DC potential obtained in the two scalae (AVE SP). Analysis of the DIF and AVE SP components has provided evidence of the multicomponent source of SP and has shown that the common assumption that SP polarity is opposite in the scala vestibuli and scala tympani is inadequate.

In ECochG, the SP recorded does not relate to either the DIF nor the AVE SP, but corresponds most closely with the SP obtained using an electrode placed within the scala tympani (Dallos, 1976). From the work of Dallos *et al.* (1972), it appears that the scala tympani SP is negative in electrical polarity when it is derived from hair cells lying on that part of the basilar membrane which corresponds to the up-slope of the travelling wave, and it is positive when obtained from hair cells activated by the down-slope of the travelling wave. This could explain the electrical polarity of the SP observed in clinical ECochG. Normally, when all the hair cells are intact, the SP is derived from hair cells closest to the round window membrane which produce an SP of negative polarity. When the hair cells within the basal turn are damaged a high frequency stimulus may elicit an SP from hair cells activated by the down-slope of the travelling wave which is positive in polarity. As the stimulus frequency is lowered, the up-slope of the travelling wave progressively lengthens until it overlies the area of remaining hair cells and so the SP polarity changes to negative (Fig. 4.6).

Békésy (1950) has shown that an upward deflection of the basilar membrane (towards the scala media) renders the scala media relatively more negative with respect to the scale tympani. Davis *et al.* (1958a) observed that the SP may reverse its polarity and become positive if the pressure in the scala tympani is raised. From these findings, one may conclude that the asymmetry normally generating a negative SP is such that the basilar membrane vibrates more upwards towards the scala media than downwards. When the pressure in the scala tympani is raised, the upward movement of the basilar membrane is limited and it vibrates more downwards than upwards. In conditions characterised by endolymphatic hydrops, the downward vibration would be limited since the

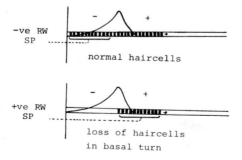

Fig. 4.6 A diagram of the mode of SP polarity obtained using a transtympanic electrode.

membrane is being stretched in this direction and so the normal up-going assymetry is enhanced, leading to a negative summating potential of increased amplitude.

The resting state potentials

The electrical potentials recorded within the cochlea may either be produced as a result of acoustic stimulation (dynamic potentials) or exist in a steady state in the absence of stimulation (static 'resting' potentials). Békésy (1952) discovered that when Reissner's membrane was pierced by a microelectrode, the potential of the endolymph within the scala media was positive with respect to an indifferent point. In the basal turn, this potential (EP) was +80 mV and 15mm further along the cochlea it was +50 mV. Tasaki, Davis and Eldredge (1954) showed that this potential was not present in the hair cells and that these possessed an intracellular potential of –60 mV (Fig. 4.7). Thus a potential difference of approximately

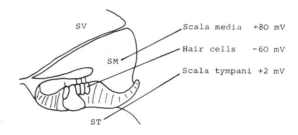

Fig. 4.7 The resting intra-cochlear potentials.

140 mV exists between the inside of the hair cell and the endolymph which surrounds it. It would appear that the EP is maintained by the stria vascularis; Tasaki and Spyropoulous (1959) have shown that the EP is greater close to this structure.

It has been found (Davis, Eldredge and Gannon., 1958b) that if the EP is increased by the introduction of a polarising current, the CM amplitude increases, and vice versa. In animals with high EP, the CM tends to be large (Wever and Vernon, 1960), so it is attractive to postulate that a piezo-electric type of change in the hair cell modifies the cell membrane permeability allowing the EP to alter the potential within the cell in a manner resembling a transistor effect. The relationship between the EP and CM is not so simple, however, as Békésy (1950) has shown that these two potentials vary quite differently with the effects of anoxia, and Butler, Konishi and Fernández (1960) have found the EP and CM alter in an unrelated manner with temperature changes. Finally, it must be noted that the EP in birds is small whilst the CM is relatively large.

The generation of nerve impulses (Fig. 4.8)

It still remains a matter of speculation exactly how the hair cell alters the mechanical energy received by its cilia into the stimulus necessary to activate the afferent nerve endings. There are some fundamental differences between the hair cells and other mechanoreceptors within the body. Cells in other parts of the body are surrounded by a fluid with high sodium and low potassium concentra-

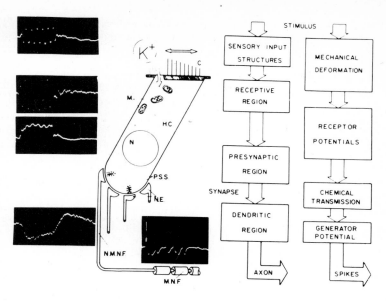

Fig. 4.8 The probable transducer mechanism of the cochlea (Dallos, P. (1975) by permission *Raven Press*).

tions and the potential difference across the cell membrane is maintained by a 'sodium pump' according to the Nernst equation. The hair cells, which contain an intracellular fluid high in potassium and low in sodium are in contact at one pole with a fluid with an almost similar composition, and tight cell junctions protect the sides of the hair cells (Beagley, 1965). It is fascinating to speculate on the functional importance of this observation; some workers have even suggested that the endolymph is not in functional contact with the hair cells. Most workers (Davis, 1961; Dallos, 1975) accept that when the cilia upon the hair cell are deformed, the electrical properties of the hair cell membrane alter, allowing electrical charge possibly related to movement of potassium ions to enter from the endolymph. This results in a positive-going change of the intracellular potential. It is possible that it is a modulation of steady potassium flux which results in the generation of the CM and some of the components of the SP (Dallos, 1975).

The electrical changes within the hair cell cause it to release a chemical transmitter which diffuses rapidly through 200 Å clefts between the hair cell bodies and the afferent endings of the cochlear nerve. The transmitter substance (probably an amino acid) causes a change in the local membrane permeability of the dendrite and results in a depolarisation termed the generator potential. Post-synaptic generator potentials have been demonstrated in the goldfish by Furu-kawa and Ishii (1967) but have not been recorded in man. It seems likely that the generator potential provides some components of the AVE SP. The generator potential is conducted along the non-myelinated segment (dendrite) of the nerve fibre and at the electrically excitable region of the fibre (probably at the habenula perforata), it excites an 'all or none' neural discharge. At the habenula perforata, the cochlear nerve becomes myelinated and it then conducts the information as a series of action potentials. It is from this region of the nerve that the AP recorded in ECochG is derived.

The action potential (AP)

The action potentials of the cochlear nerve may be either recorded directly from the nerve or individual nerve fibres, or after conduction through the cochlear fluids from the round window or a more distant site. The AP recorded during electrocochleography is the sum of many individual AP along a length of the basilar membrane. Some workers prefer to use the term 'whole-nerve action potential' (WN AP) when the AP is evoked by a click as evidence suggests that it represents neural activity from the whole length of the basilar membrane. The term WN AP is not appropriate when a frequency specific stimulus is used as under these circumstances only a limited length of the basilar membrane is activated and the term 'compound action potential' (C AP) is suggested.

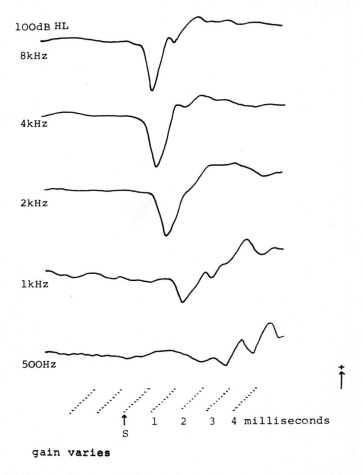

Fig. 4.9 Compound action potentials obtained using various short tone burst stimuli.

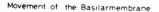

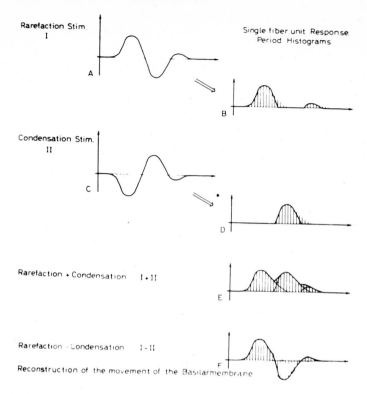

Fig. 4.10 Imaginary curves of movement of the basilar membrane and related single fibre unit response-period histograms for a 500 Hz stimulus (Elberling, C. & Salomon, G. (1971), by permission *Revue de Laryngologie*).

It is found, as expected, that the greater the number of individual nerve fibres firing in synchrony, the larger and more readily identifiable is the AP. A click is known to stimulate the whole of the basilar membrane and, indeed, Elberling (1976c) has shown how the potential recorded can be analysed according to the velocity of the travelling wave to yield frequency information. Frequency selective masking experiments, however, reveal that the major contribution to the click-evoked AP is derived from the basal turn of the cochlea (Teas, Eldredge and Davis, 1962). There are two explanations for this finding. Firstly, the travelling wave is progressively damped as it travels along the basilar membrane towards the apex (Zwicker and Fastl, 1972). This presupposes that the number of hair cells firing in a given section of the basilar membrane depends on the degree of displacement. Secondly, the velocity of the propogation of the travelling wave slows markedly as it approaches the apex of the cochlea and this results in a decrease in the number of hair cells firing per unit time (Zerlin, 1969).

Pure tone bursts of short duration can be used to evoke the AP and the latency of the AP then directly reflects the speed of the travelling wave (Fig. 4.9). High frequency tone bursts (above 2 000 Hz) evoke an excellent AP as their onset is abrupt and they stimulate the relevant area of the basilar membrane with reasonable synchrony. Lower frequency tone bursts (1 000–500 Hz) do evoke a frequency specific AP but this AP becomes progressively smaller, broader and more prolonged as the frequency is lowered. At frequencies of 250 Hz or less, the AP is practically unidentifiable. The problems involved in evoking low frequency AP are now discussed using the 500 Hz tone burst as an example.

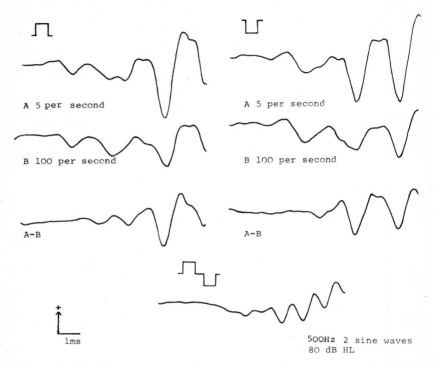

Fig. 4.11 The ECochG recordings of a 500 Hz compound action potential showing the effect of reversing the polarity of the stimulus by half a cycle.

At 500 Hz, the stimulus has a slow rise time which in itself argues against synchronisation. Furthermore, the travelling wave which reaches the apical turn of the cochlea is damped and of a slow velocity. The phase of the stimulating wave must also be considered. Brugge *et al*. (1969) have shown that an AP is only generated when the basilar membrane moves in an upward direction. Elberling and Salomon (1971) have constructed a model of the basilar membrane movement in response to a 500 Hz stimulus (Fig. 4.10). It may be seen that if the AP is obtained in the usual manner by alternately inverting the phase of the stimulus (to remove CM), the average of the 500 Hz AP is the sum of at least three separately evoked AP (Fig. 4.11).

Altering the intensity of stimulation affects the amplitude, latency and configuration of the whole nerve AP (Fig. 4.12). At high intensities (110 dB HL)

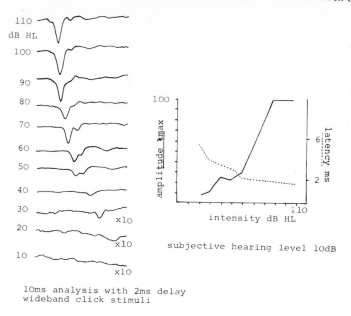

10ms analysis with 2ms delay
wideband click stimuli

Fig. 4.12 The whole-nerve (click) action potentials of a normally-hearing subject and the amplitude and intensity versus stimulus intensity (input/output) graph.

the AP has three negative peaks and the positive peak following the N1 does not usually overshoot the baseline by any great extent. In these circumstances the N1 is said to be 'monophasic' and its latency (timing between the arrival of the stimulus at the tympanic membrane and the peak of N1) is in the order of 1.2 ms. As the stimulus intensity decreases the amplitude of the AP diminishes until at about 50–60 dB HL a temporary plateau is reached. This plateau remains for a few dB and then, as the stimulus intensity falls below 40–50 dB HL, the amplitude again diminishes until the response is no longer identifiable at about 10 dB HL (close to the subjective hearing threshold). The amplitude/intensity function may therefore be separated into 'H' (High) and 'L' (Low) areas (Yoshie, 1968). It is interesting that patients with recruiting hearing disorders often appear to have lost the 'L' part of the graph. The latency of the AP increases gradually as the stimulus intensity diminishes until the amplitude plateau is reached and at this point the latency changes more rapidly. Examination of the waveform of the normal AP shows that at high intensities it is the N1 which predominates but at around 50–60 dB HL the response become 'W' shaped as the N2 component becomes equal in amplitude to the N1. At lower stimulus intensities the N2 appears to be the only discernible component and it is this part of the AP which is traced to low stimulus levels.

There are three theories to account for the shape and intensity functions of the compound AP. Perhaps the true explanation takes all these theories into account.

Hypothesis I. The first explanation of the shape of the normal AP at different intensities depends on the pattern of innervation of the inner and outer hair cells. Teas *et al*. (1962) have stated that the complexity of the AP results from the summation of asynchronous nerve action potentials each possessing a diphasic waveform. The AP can be explained as the sum of two partly overlapping Gausian distribution functions (Eggermont and Spoor, 1973a). A simplified diagram is shown in Figure 4.13. These statements suggest the presence of two different populations of afferent nerve fibres; population I predominating at high intensity levels over 60–70 dB, and population II predominating at intensity levels below 30 dB. At one time it was thought that these two populations were the radial and spiral afferent nerve fibres.

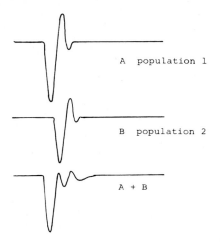

Fig. 4.13 A simple explanation for the shape of the whole-nerve action potential based on the theory of two nerve fibre populations.

The inner hair cells are mainly innervated by radial fibres. These hair cells are situated towards the edge of the basilar membrane and away from the site of maximum displacement. A low intensity stimulus may only vibrate the centre of the basilar membrane sufficiently to cause outer hair cell stimulation, and the inner hair cells may not be excited until the stimulus intensity is raised. The radial afferent fibres outnumber the spiral fibres by a ratio of 20 : 1 (Spoendlin, 1966); this implies that in the case of a linear increase in amplitude of the compound AP with the number of nerve fibres activated, the maximum output of the two populations should differ also by a ratio of 20 : 1. This is exactly what is observed by electrocochleography at high stimulus intensity levels. So it was concluded that at high intensities, the N1 originates mostly from the inner hair cells and that the 'H' part of the intensity/amplitude graph reflects the activity of these hair cells.

The N2 component of the compound AP at high stimulus intensities can be traced down to the psychophysical threshold and appears to be the only potential recorded at stimulus intensities of less than 30–40 dB SL. This part of the AP is identified, therefore, with the outer hair cells and is responsible for the 'L' part of the intensity/amplitude graph. The longer latency of the N2, compared with the

N1, may be due to a delay along the non-myelinated dendrites of the spiral fibres; this delay is much longer than that of the radial fibres. The antibiotic streptomycin damages the outer hair cells specifically and Stange, Spreng and Kiedel (1964) have shown that, in these circumstances, the 'H' part of the graph is essentially unaltered whilst the 'L' part of the graph is absent. Similar findings have been reported by Kiang, Moxon and Levine (1970) using Kanamycin.

Hypothesis II.   The main argument against the first hypothesis results from the finding, using single fibre recording techniques, that the cochlear nerve, central to the spiral ganglion, is relatively homogenous in terms of its constituent fibre threshold and filtering properties (Kiang, 1968; Evans, 1972). There is no evidence from properly controlled recent experiments to suggest that there are two populations of fibres which can be distinguished on a threshold basis.

The technique of single fibre recordings is well described by Evans (1972). Basically, after suitable preparation of the animal, a microelectrode is placed into the cochlear nerve within the internal acoustic meatus and delicately manipulated into a single fibre. Tone bursts are delivered at a rate of 4–5 per second and the neural discharges occurring at varying stimulus intensities as the stimulus frequency is swept from high– low– high are plotted by a computer (*see* Fig. 4.3). The frequency tuning curve (FTC) for a single fibre is sharp at minimum intensities, indicating the characteristic frequency (CF) of that fibre, and then broadens moderately as the stimulus intensity increases, until at

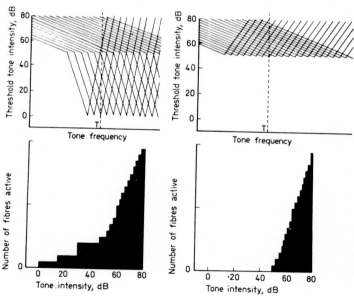

Fig. 4.14 A schematic diagram illustrating the rate of growth in the number of active cochlear fibres with increasing stimulus intensity level in normal (left) and abnormal, recruiting (right) cochleae. Tone indicated by dashed line at T. Upper diagrams show the tuning curves of single cochlear fibres. Lower diagrams show the growth in number of active fibres. These lower diagrams can be compared to the input/output functions shown in figures 4.12 and 4.26 (Evans, E.G. (1975b), by permission *Audiology*).

approximately 60 dB SL the shoulders of the tuning curve become markedly widened in the low frequency direction. Evans (1975a) describes a model based on these observations which accounts for the amplitude/intensity graph of the AP in ECochG (Fig. 4.14). At low intensities, the AP is derived from those neural units lying within the tip of the overlapping tuning curves and this corresponds with the 'L' portion of the graph. At stimulus intensities in excess of 60 dB SL, the AP is formed from units firing within the broad portion of the tuning curves and, as many more units contribute, this corresponds to the 'H' portion of the graph. A rather similar model has also been proposed by Ödzamer and Dallos (1976). Evans (1975a) further suggests that if the cochlea is anoxic or damaged by an ototoxic antibiotic, only the broad parts of the tuning curves remain so that the amplitude/intensity functions of the AP correspond only to the 'H' portion of the graph.

Tuning curves can be obtained using electrocochleography (Dallos and Cheatham, 1976). The AP is elicited using a tone and then the response is masked using a second tone (tone on tone masking). The bandwidth of the second tone necessary to mask completely the AP response is recorded at each intensity until the tuning curve has been obtained. Eggermont (1976) has obtained compound AP tuning curves in man and his results are in close agreement with the previous animal studies.

The finding that all the individual fibres of the cochlear nerve display the same intensity threshold requires an explanation since the outer hair cells are more sensitive to minimal intensities than the inner hair cells. There is no evidence of synaptic contact or branching between the radial and spiral fibres within the cochlea or within the spiral ganglion (Smith and Dempsey, 1957; Spoendlin, 1976). Evans (1975b) proposes an excitation theory; the activity generated within the spiral fibre by the outer hair cell generates sufficient local current to activate nearby radial fibres. Zwislocki (1974, 1975) proposes an inhibitory theory; the output of the outer hair cells acting as a means of sharpening the tuning of the inner hair cells. At present, both these theories have merit but neither has yet been substantiated by direct evidence.

Hypothesis III.   The tuning curves explain the amplitude/intensity functions of the AP but not its shape and latency. The shape of the WN AP is a result of a complex integration, or convolution, of the unit activity along the length of the cochlea, where separate units possess different time delays, thresholds and possibly polarities (Teas *et al.*, 1962; Elberling, 1973, 1974, 1976b, 1976c). The basal coil of the cochlea contains the neural elements which fire with the greatest degree of synchrony and it appears that the N1 of the WN AP reflects the activity of this area. Neural elements further along the cochlear partition fire with less synchrony and with a longer latency according to the speed of the travelling wave, and so add in a complex manner to form the later parts of the WN AP waveform.

The contributions to the WN AP from various segments of the basilar membrane may be *derived* using a high pass masking technique (Teas *et al.*, 1962). This technique may be described by the following example: a click stimulus is delivered which stimulates the whole of the cochlea and a high pass noise is presented simultaneously masking all the frequencies above 2 kHz, with a steep 'cut-off' of 60–100 dB per octave. The response to this situation is stored (store B). Next the same click stimulus is delivered but the high pass noise now masks all frequencies above 4 kHz and the response is stored (store A). The computer finally subtracts the response in store B from the response in store A and the result is the derived AP for the cochlear segment from 2–4 kHz.

Elberling (1973, 1974) has investigated extensively the manner in which derived AP for different cochlear segments can be added together (convolution) to create the waveform of the WN AP (Fig. 4.15). He postulates that as the intensity of the click is decreased, the increase in latency of the WN AP is related to the derivation of the response from successively more apical parts of the cochlea. By modelling the manner in which the derived AP convolute to form the WN AP, he has devised a method of deconvoluting a WN AP obtained from a patient so that the relative contributions from each segment of the cochlea can be determined (Elberling, 1976c). This method can be used to estimate the pure tone audiogram from WN AP recordings.

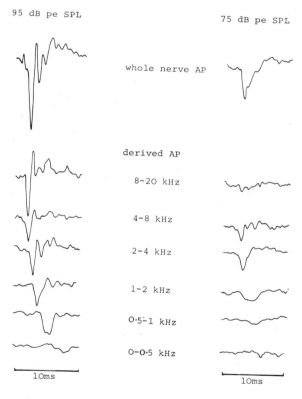

Fig. 4.15 Whole-nerve action potential recordings and derived action potential curves at 95 dB p.e. SPL (left) and 75 dB p.e. SPL (right) in a normally-hearing subject. (As the individual action potential curves are based on differences between two masked action potential recordings containing unaffected cochlear microphonic, this latter potential is not present in the derived curves) (Adapted from Elberling, C. (1974)).

The compound AP for pure tone stimuli at high intensities is also a result of the convolution of neural elements from a length of the cochlear partition (Elberling, 1976b) but this area becomes much more limited as the intensity of the stimulus decreases. At low stimulus intensities, the C AP becomes more frequency specific.

In conclusion, it may be seen that there is merit to all three hypotheses mentioned. The 'L' part of the amplitude/intensity graph does probably indicate the functional integrity of the outer hair cells. The FTC do provide an adequate explanation for the amplitude changes of the AP in normal and pathological cases, and finally the concept of convolution of the individual unit contributions along the cochlea partition does answer some of the remaining questions regarding the latency and waveform.

Some characteristics of the responses

The electrode positions

The AP may be recorded from various sites around the head (promontory, tympanic membrane, ear canal, ear lobe, scalp, hard palate, nasopharynx, etc.). The electrical activity passes relatively less freely through the more resistant tissues such as bone. Inevitably, the closer the active electrode is placed to the round window, the larger the potentials recorded. The threshold of activity of the cochlear neurones is obviously independent of the site of the electrode and so, in theory are the thresholds obtained from the more distant sites – unless swamped by background electrical activity. Yoshie (1973) has remarked that the AP threshold is on average 17.6 dB lower when recorded directly from the promontory rather than the ear canal.

Eggermont and Odenthal (1974b) have presented the following data after reviewing the literature:

1. The amplitude of promontory AP to high intensities of stimulation is 10–30 μV pp (peak to peak value).
2. The amplitude of promontory AP to 10 dB SL stimuli is 0.2 μV pp.
3. The amplitude of ear canal AP to high intensities of stimulation is 1–2 μV pp.
4. The amplitude of ear canal AP to 10 dB SL stimuli is 0.1 μV pp.

Further consideration of the current literature reveals:

5. The amplitude of mastoid or ear lobe AP (N1 of BER) to high intensities of stimulation is 0.6–1.1 μV pp.
6. The amplitude of mastoid or ear lobe AP to 40 dB SL stimuli is 0.05–0.1 μV pp.

It is not usually possible to identify the AP from mastoid or ear lobe recordings at levels of less than 40 dB SL as the responses cannot be differentiated from the background activity or noise (Thornton, 1975a).

Examination of this data reveals that the attenuation varies with the intensity of stimulation in each case and that the low intensity evoked AP travels relatively more easily to distant sites than the high intensity evoked AP. The ability to detect the AP at threshold levels depends on the level of background activity and the extent to which this may be negated by averaging techniques. Elberling (1976a) has estimated the background noise at each site:

A. The background noise level for promontory recordings is approximately 6.8 μV pp.

B. The background noise level for ear canal recordings (with the electrode embedded in the meatal skin) is 3.4 μV. pp

C. The background noise level for ear lobe recordings is 20.3 μV pp.

The level of the background noise depends both on the impedance between the electrode and the underlying tissues and on the ability of the active and reference electrodes to receive potentials from extraneous sources (e.g. muscle, EEG, etc.). The promontory electrode has a high impedance of approximately 60 kΩ but, with the reference electrode placed on the ipsilateral ear lobe, little extraneous noise is encountered. The electrode embedded in the external acoustic meatal skin has a low input impedance, probably less than 3 kΩ, and is placed almost as favourably as the promontory electrode as regards extraneous noise. An ear canal electrode which does not penetrate the tissues has a far higher input impedance approaching that of the promontory electrode and picks up much more noise. The ear lobe or mastoid electrode may have a low input impedance but with the reference placed on the vertex a considerable amount of background noise is included in the recordings.

The waveform and functions of the AP recorded from the ear canal are essentially identical to those from promontory recordings although there may be some minor difference due to a low frequency filtering effect occurring as the response passes through the more resistant tissues (Elberling, 1976a). The functions of the AP recorded from the ear lobe or mastoid are similar and often reveal the 'H' and 'L' areas of the amplitude/intensity graph. Often a high level for the high pass filter is chosen (250–500 Hz) which alters the AP waveform (see Fig. 4.19).

There is reason for optimism that eventually a technique will be developed which will avoid the need to penetrate the tympanic membrane or lining of the meatus with the active electrode. Until then, the clearest recordings continue to be obtained by these somewhat invasive approaches.

Effect of prolonged or repeated stimulation (habituation)

The amplitude, latency and waveform of the AP is constant despite prolonged or repeated stimulation and no evidence of habituation has been obtained. Providing that the electrode is replaced accurately, these functions remain remarkably constant from day to day within the same individual. The CM and SP, since neither are neural potentials, are not affected by habituation. The CM, however, changes dramatically with even slight alterations in the positioning of the electrode on the promontory.

Effect of stimulus presentation rates (equilibration)

Eggermont and Spoor (1973a) give an excellent description of the results of equilibration (adaptation) experiments in guinea pigs. Their findings appear to

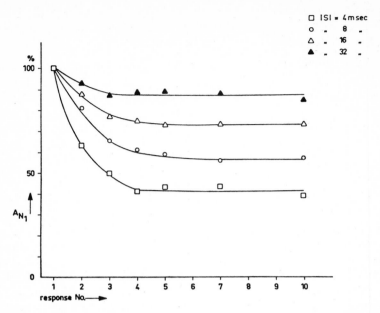

Fig. 4.16 The relative amplitude (AN1) of the N1 deflection of the compound action potential as a function of the response number at different interstimulus interval (ISI) values and at a SPL of 30 dB (Eggermont, J.J. & Spoor, A. (1973a), by permission *Audiology*).

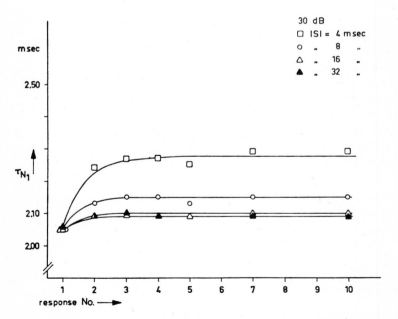

Fig. 4.17 The latency (τN1) of the N1 deflection of the compound action potential as a function of the response number at different ISI values and at a SPL of 30 dB (Eggermont, J.J. & Spoor, A. (1973a), by permission *Audiology*).

apply closely to human physiology. They found that decreasing the interstimulus interval (ISI) altered the amplitude, latency and waveform of the AP but had no noticeable effect on the CM and SP. The ISI is a measure of the time elapsing between the end of one stimulus and the beginning of the next. The stimulus rate is the number of stimuli delivered, usually per second. One can only relate the ISI and stimulus rate if one knows the length of the stimulus—for example: ISI 200 ms, stimulus length 50 ms, stimulus rate four per second. These effects are due to the fact that the AP depends on the firing of individual nerve fibres and that each nerve fibre requires a short recovery period after each firing (refractory period) before another neural impulse may be initiated. The equilibrium value for any of the functions at a given ISI interval is generally reached after 5 stimuli, and after this period the pattern of firing of individual fibres reaches a steady state. The findings of Eggermont and Spoor (1973a) are as follows:

1. The amplitude of the AP remains at approximately 100 per cent of its value for rates up to 7 per second (ISI, approximately 140 ms) and only alters fractionally at rates up to 14 per second (ISI, approximately 70 ms). Figure 4.16 shows the reduction in the amplitude of the N1 component of the AP (A N1) at faster ISI intervals.

2. The latency of the N1 (τ N1) component of the AP increases with shorter ISI (Fig. 4.17). This property of the AP has to be considered when subtraction techniques at different repetition rates are used to extract the AP from the SP.

3. The width of the N1 ($\triangle$ N1) component of the AP increases in a manner fully comparable to the increase in latency (τ N1) (Fig. 4.18).

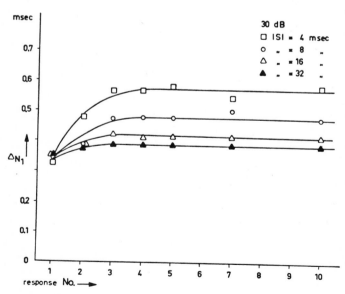

Fig. 4.18 The width ($\triangle$ N1) of the N1 deflection of the compound action potential as a function of the response number at different ISI values and at a SPL of 30 dB (Eggermont, J.J. & Spoor, A. (1973a), by permission *Audiology*).

Effect of masking (random) noise

Eggermont and Spoor (1973b) also describe the effects of continuous masking noise on the AP. The mechanism by which masking affects the amplitude, latency and width of the AP is the same as that responsible for adaptation. In effect the masking noise fires the nerve fibres at a maximum rate and does not allow them a sufficient refractory period. Coats (1964a; 1964b; 1967; 1971) has made detailed studies and the reader is referred to these works for further information.

The effect of masking is especially important when electrocochleography is performed in areas which are not sound-proofed. The low frequencies, especially, are easily masked, making threshold information impossible in noisy circumstances.

Effect of sedation

Fortunately sedatives, including general anaesthetic agents, appear to have no effect on the functions of the cochlear responses (AP, CM, SP). This property greatly enhances the value of ECochG in testing young children who cannot be relied on to co-operate whilst awake.

Frequency specificity of the responses

The CM obtained by transtympanic ECochG is not frequency specific as it only relates to a small area of the basilar membrane close to the round window.

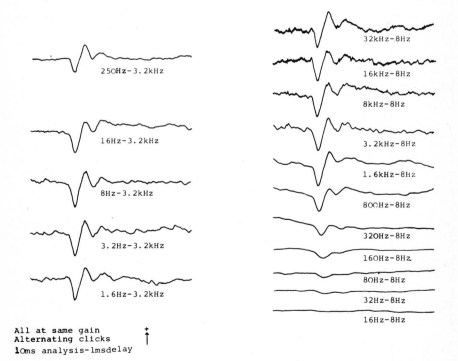

Fig. 4.19 The effect of limiting the system bandwidth on the whole-nerve action potential.

The hair cells in this position respond to all frequencies but give the largest CM amplitudes to low frequency stimuli. (The lower the frequency, the larger the area of the basilar membrane moving in approximately the same phase.).

Tone bursts are excellent stimuli for evoking compound AP at specific frequencies. The problems attached to the use of these stimuli have been discussed earlier in this chapter. They evoke a compound AP which is certainly specific for frequencies between 1 kHz and 8 kHz, especially at stimulus intensities below 65 dB HL (Eggermont and Odenthal, 1974a) and accurate estimations of the audiometric threshold may be made at these frequencies.

At stimulus levels above 65 dB HL, the AP evoked by a tone burst is altered by bandstop masking at the same frequency (Eggermont and Odenthal, 1974a). The explanation is that all the units lying within the broad area of the FTC are contributing to the response. Some reservation must be made therefore when discussing the frequency specificity for these higher stimulus intensities until further work has been completed.

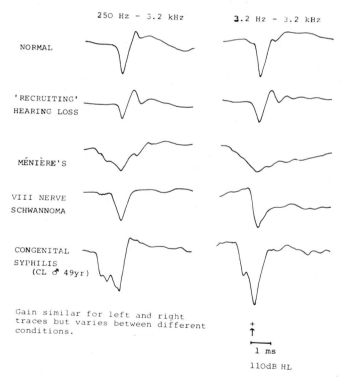

Fig. 4.20 The effect of limiting the system bandwidth on the characteristic action potential waveforms encountered in certain pathological conditions (Ramsden, R.T., Moffat, D.A. & Gibson, W.P.R. (1977), by permission *Annals of Otology, Rhinology and Laryngology*).

Effect of altering bandwidth recording limits

Analysis of the AP reveals that the majority of the energy lies between 600 Hz and 1.2 kHz, but there are contributions from outside this frequency range. The use of too high a setting for the high pass filter (HPF) leads to a differentiation of the normal AP which appears sharper and more diphasic. The effect of recording the AP from a patient with a 40 dB HL 'cochlear' hearing loss using various bandwidths is shown in Figure 4.19.

The recording of low frequency contributions to the AP is especially important in abnormal cases. Figure 4.20 shows several examples. The classic broad waveform of the AP obtained from a patient with an eighth nerve tumour may be completely lost if too high an HPF setting is used. The usual bandwidth limits for ECochG are approximately 3.2 Hz to 3.2 kHz although the exact settings do vary at different laboratories.

The SP is essentially a DC response and ideally a very low HPF should be used. Nevertheless, worthwhile recordings of SP are obtained using HPF settings of 3.2 Hz or more.

Crosstalk

No AP can be recorded from the promontory or ear canal of the deaf ear of a patient with a unilateral hearing loss. This absence of crosstalk is a most valuable property for it allows an accurate estimation of cochlear function to be made without the need for any masking whatsoever. Even using ear lobe or mastoid electrodes (BER), the N1 (equivalent to the action potential in ECochG) cannot be recorded from the contralateral ear although there is considerable crossover of the later waves.

Masking of the contralateral ear does have an effect on the AP, presumably due to the action of the efferent olivo-cochlear bundle (Galambos, 1956b; Desmedt, 1962). Clinically, this field has not yet been exploited and awaits further investigation.

The test and test/retest reliability

The test reliability of ECochG is better than any of the other tests mentioned in this book. The agreement between the AP threshold and the psychoacoustic threshold is close. Tone bursts evoke compound AP (CAP) which may be used to estimate the pure tone audiogram (PTA). For frequencies of 2 kHz or higher, the difference between the CAP threshold and the PTA threshold is usually less than 10 dB (Aran *et al.*, 1971). The author has reviewed 40 recordings from adults with normal hearing or with sensory or conductive hearing losses. The CAP threshold, using stimulus frequencies of 2 kHz, 4 kHz and 8 kHz, was within −5 to +10 dB of the PTA threshold in 85 per cent of the subjects, and the remainder were within +10 to +25 dB. The impression was gained that the correlation was the least favourable in subjects with conductive hearing losses but there was not sufficient data to allow statistical analysis.

At lower frequencies, the correlation between the PTA and ECochG is less exact. Antonelli (1976) tested 39 adults and evoked a just detectable CAP in 75 per cent of subjects at 0–10 dB SL. The author has examined recordings from 30 subjects, the 1 kHz CAP threshold was within 0 to +20 dB of the 1 kHz PTA threshold in 80 per cent of cases and within 0 to +40 dB in all cases. In the author's experience, the correlation between the CAP and PTA at 500 Hz was poor with the gap amounting to 60 dB in some cases. The author has not been able to recognise a CAP at 250 Hz even at 100 dB SL in more than a handful of subjects. It may be concluded that the ECochG provides a reliable indication of the PTA only in the higher audiometric frequencies.

The test/retest reliability of ECochG is excellent. The waveform and latency of the AP is remarkably constant even when recorded at intervals of several weeks. The amplitude of the AP does vary between test sessions, as the amplitude is altered by small changes in both the electrode position and electrode impedance. The excellent test/retest reliability of the AP makes it a useful tool for assessing the changes that may occur within the cochlea after medical or surgical treatment.

The CM does not vary providing the electrode position and electrode impedance are not altered. If the active electrode is reinserted, changes in both amplitude and phase may occur. The phase of the CM alters dramatically when the electrode tip is positioned at different sites around the round window niche.

Instrumentation

The apparatus required for ECochG is basically that described in Chapter Two. The author uses the Medelec/Amplaid Mk III equipment but those understanding electronics better, such as engineers and physicists, may prefer the greater adaptability of apparatus they assemble themselves. The special requirements for ECochG are listed over the next few pages.

The test environment

Subjects are best tested lying relaxed upon a couch. The test chamber must be large enough to accomodate the couch and an operating microscope for accurate placement of the electrode. If children are tested under Ketamine ® or similar anaesthetic drugs, suction apparatus should be readily to hand. Some workers prefer general inhalation anaesthetic agents; Hutton (1976) has described the necessary arrangements for venting the expired gases outside the test chamber using an Enderby valve.

The room must be sound proof if accurate threshold estimations are to be made. Background noise within the test area interferes particularly with the measurement of the compound AP at low stimulus frequencies. When adults are tested for neuro-otological purposes, the need for sound proofing is not so great. Ideally, the room should be anechoic.

The stimulus generation

Stimulus requirements.   These have already been mentioned. In summary, the AP is obtained using very brief stimuli with relatively sharp onset characteristics. Clicks of 70–100 μs evoke the whole nerve AP. Filtered clicks with onset transients have not proved to be frequency specific. Tone bursts elicit frequency specific, compound AP but sharp onsets may produce click artefacts; Eggermont and Odenthal (1974a) recommend stimuli of six sine waves—two sine waves rise time, two sine waves plateau and two sine waves decay.

Stimulus repetition rates.   The stimulus repetition rate used clinically is often a compromise between the adaptation of the AP resulting from fast rates and the time taken to accumulate sufficient individual responses (epochs) to yield a clear-cut averaged AP. Most workers use a rate of 10 per second which is ideal for neuro-otological work. A stimulus repetition rate of 20 per second is convenient for threshold estimations, as this shortens the period of testing.

At stimulus intensity levels above 40 dB SL, 128 epochs yield a clear response. At levels close to threshold, up to 512 epochs may be necessary.

Stimulus transducer.   Either a loudspeaker or an earphone may be used. Unless the test chamber is anechoic, the stimulus delivered by a loudspeaker will echo back to the test ear after bouncing off walls, etc., and evoke further responses. An earphone is better but should be enclosed in mu-metal to prevent the recording of electromagnetic artefacts which may contaminate recordings of the CM. A closed acoustic system is ideal and may be used if the method advocated by Elberling and Salomon (1971) is employed.

Stimulus calibration.   The brief stimuli used during ECochG may be calibrated in peak equivalent SPL terms. Most clinicians prefer a physiological calibration (dB HL) as this is more easily compared with the 'subjective' pure tone audiogram. Further details are given in Chapter 2.

The stimulus intensity is usually graduated in 5 dB steps.

Masking facilities.   These are not required for clinical testing but are useful to the research worker.

The recording equipment

The electrodes.   The type of electrode used varies considerably with the method used for recording the ECochG.

1. Transtympanic ECochG: A thin steel wire of approximately 0.3mm diameter, insulated except for the very tip and the opposite end at which it makes contact with the electrode holder, is commonly used (Fig. 4.21). The best electrode holder is a screw-type of arrangement which grips the electrode firmly, the free end being notched to receive the elastic from the ear surround which holds the electrode gently in place.

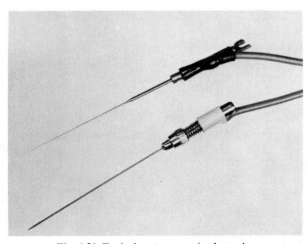

Fig. 4.21 Typical transtympanic electrodes.

2. Extratympanic ECochG: The surface electrode usually rests on the posterior-inferior rim of the drum. The wire should be flexible enough to prevent any possibility of the electrode being driven through the tympanic membrane but firm enough to remain in the desired position.

Electrodes which pierce the surface of the meatus yield better responses as the electrode/tissue impedance is much lower. Some workers (e.g. Coats and Dickey, 1970) use a wire electrode, similar to that used for transtympanic testing. Elberling and Salomon (1971) use a more complex technique for positioning the electrode which is more convenient during the test period. They pierce the posterior meatal wall with a hypodermic syringe needle at a position immediately behind the pinna and then insert a silver wire. The hypodermic needle is then removed and the silver wire electrode is accurately embedded into the meatal lining at a point close to the postero-inferior rim of the meatus. Not only does this method give stability but it allows the use of an entirely closed acoustic system.

Amplifiers. Low noise biological amplifiers are essential with a high input impedance and a high common mode rejection. The total gain required varies from 10^4 to 10^6. Usually a preamplifier with a fixed gain is positioned close to the patient and the final gain adjustment is made by altering the settings on the main amplifier housed with the averager.

Filter settings (system bandwidth). Most clinical workers use a system bandwidth which varies from 2–10 Hz (HPF) and from 3–5 kHz (HPF). The effect of altering the bandwidth on the AP was shown in Figures 4.19 and 4.20.

The averager. Any properly programmed computer may be used and small purpose-built averagers (e.g. Medelec DAV6) are adequate. Usually a 10 ms analysis time is employed with a minimum of 20 memory addresses per millisecond to allow adequate resolution of the potentials.

The monitor oscilloscope. It is helpful but not essential to monitor the on-going unaveraged signal during each recording as occasionally artefacts may occur which might lead to misinterpretation of the responses. At near threshold levels, it is convenient to watch the averaged response building so that any inconsistencies may be detected.

Artefact rejection facilities. It is advantageous to have a means of automatically rejecting any sudden high voltage artefacts which may occur. Details are given in Chapter Two.

Permanent recordings of the results. These are essential, especially in neuro-otological work so that the responses may be analysed in detail after the test period. Various methods are available and these are discussed in Chapter Two. Timing details and a calibration pulse revealing the amplitude of a set voltage should be included on every set of permanent recordings. Most clinical workers now record a negative potential as a downward deflection although electrophysiologists may prefer to retain the standard of recording negative potential as an upgoing deflection. Whichever polarity is used, it must be clearly stated on the recordings.

Testing procedures

Transtympanic electrocochleography. Children under the age of 12 years are generally tested under general anaesthetia, whilst adults may be tested using local anaesthesia.

General anaesthesia is usually administered by a trained anaesthetist and full regard is given to safety. Ketamine ® is favoured by many clinics but should not be given to older children or adults as it may cause unpleasant hallucinations. Hutton (1976) recommends a dosage of 1mg IM for each 35 cm² of body surface area. (The surface area may be calculated from the height (H) and the weight (W) of the patient by the Du Bois formula: Surface area $= W^0.^{425} \times H^0.^{725} \times 71.84$, where W is recorded in kg and H is recorded in cm). Inhalation anaesthesia may be used but care must be taken to vent the expired gases outside the close confines of the test chamber.

Local anaesthesia is not essential and satisfactory work may be performed without anaesthesia. Some workers spray the tympanic membrane with local anaesthetic such as Cetacaine ® but it is doubtful whether this substance actually penetrates the squamous epithelium. A much more satisfactory technique involves the iontophoresis of the local anaesthetic agent driving it into the drum. This method is virtually painless except for some slight discomfort experienced by a few patients when the electrode touches the promontory (Ramsden, Gibson and Moffat, 1977). Whichever method is used to place the electrode, the discomfort is minimal. Certainly no patient has ever asked to defer the testing of the second ear and most have remarked that the test was less unpleasant than the standard Hallpike-FitzGerald caloric test. Some workers give the subject a small dose of a sedative such as Valium ® prior to the test period.

Extra-tympanic electrocochleography. Insertion of electrodes in the meatal wall is usually preceded by an injection of a local anaesthetic agent such as Lignocaine. The post-auricular branch of the Vagus nerve supplies this part of the meatus and may be blocked by an injection placed at the midpoint of the

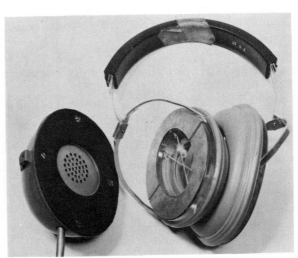

Fig. 4.22 The shielded earphone and headring assembly used for transtympanic electrocochleography.

posterior meatal wall. Surface techniques have the advantage that no discomfort is involved and so no anaesthesia is necessary.

Electrode stabilisation.   The transtympanic electrode is usually secured in position by a ring placed firmly around the ear (Fig. 4.22) and the electrode is held against the promontory by gentle pressure afforded by elastic thread attached to this ring. Surface electrodes are often secured by adhesive glue at the external opening of the meatus.

Electrode positions.   The earth electrode is usually a standard EEG silver/silver chloride electrode disc placed on the forehead. The reference electrode is either a similar electrode or a clip electrode placed on the ear lobe of the test ear. It is not necessary to make great efforts to lower the electrode/skin resistance of these electrodes when using either transtympanic electrocochleography and levels under $10k\Omega$ are acceptable.

The active electrode for promontory recording is placed through the tympanic membrane at a point midway between the postero-inferior rim of the annulus and the umbo. This manoeuvre must be done expertly by a medically-trained person. It is wise to reassure the unanaesthetised patient by saying something on these lines: 'I am now going to touch the lower part of the ear with a wire. You may feel this but please do not move as any discomfort is only momentary. The wire will touch the lowest part of the ear where it is safe'. If the patient has a hearing loss, it is essential to make sure he has understood this message so that he does not jerk his head.

Extratympanic recordings are made after placing the active electrode as close to the postero-inferior rim of the tympanic membrane as possible.

Identification of the responses

The identification of the AP at intensities of 40 dB SL or above is a simple matter. The latency is approximately 1.2 to 2 ms. The CM and SP are similarly easy to identify. The ease of identification of the responses is one of the main attractions of this method of ERA.

Isolation of the AP.   The AP is the most useful potential obtained by ECochG as it provides an accurate measure of the threshold of cochlear function

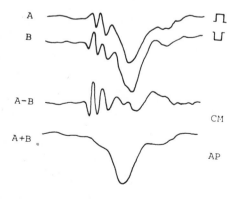

Fig. 4.23 An illustration of separation of the cochlear microphonic and action potential (and summating potential) by using the technique of alternately reversing the phase of the stimulus.

and as the waveform of the AP complex may be characteristic in certain pathological conditions.

The AP may be conveniently isolated by alternately reversing the phase of the acoustic stimulus during averaging. The CM alters phase in keeping with the alteration of the phase of the stimulus, so that the sum of the CM to an equal number of condensation and rarefaction stimuli is approximately zero (Fig. 4.23). The AP always occurs as a negative potential regardless of the phase of the stimulus and the sum of the AP evoked by rarefaction and condensation stimuli is an AP of approximately twice the size of the AP evoked by a single stimulus. Elberling and Salomon (1971) have stressed that rarefaction and condensation phases of the same stimulus do not evoke a similar AP particularly at low frequencies (see Fig. 4.10). The AP evoked by alternating phases of stimulation represents the mean of the two waveforms. Using high frequency and click stimulation, the CM is usually small in amplitude at intensity levels below 70 dB SL and some workers feel that it is unnecessary to continue alternating the phase of the stimulus at these intensity levels. Certainly if one is attempting to isolate the 500 Hz AP at near threshold levels, it is an advantage not to alternate the starting phase of the stimulus as this leads to blurring of the response. If the CM is troublesome, it can be removed by another subtraction technique. First, the

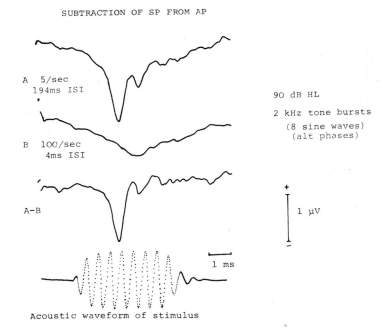

SUBTRACTION OF SP FROM AP

A   5/sec
194ms ISI

B   100/sec
4ms ISI

A-B

Acoustic waveform of stimulus

90 dB HL

2 kHz tone bursts
(8 sine waves)
(alt phases)

+

1 µV

1 ms

Fig. 4.24 An illustration of removal of the summating potential (SP) contribution of the AP/SP complex. A shows SP and AP of maximum amplitude evoked by stimuli presented five times each second (long ISI). B shows SP and an AP of reduced amplitude due to equilibration as the stimuli were presented 100 times each second (short ISI). Subtracting A from B (A-B) removes the SP component completely as it has the same amplitude on traces A and B, and leaves the AP visible. This AP represents the difference between the maximal AP in store A and the equilibrated AP in store B.

response is obtained with a long interstimulus interval (ISI) (10 stimuli/second) and stored (store A). Next, the response is obtained using the same stimulus but at a very short ISI (100 stimuli/second) and the response is stored (store B). Finally, subtraction of the responses in each store (A–B) reveals the AP alone removing any CM and SP contributions.

Isolation of CM. The CM is helpful in clinical ECochG, although it does arise from only a limited area of the basilar membrane close to the round window; it is not directly related to the threshold of cochlear function and it is not frequency specific.

The CM may be isolated by using alternating phases of stimulation and by subtracting the result of one phase (e.g. condensation) from the opposite phase (e.g. rarefaction). In this manner the CM obtained in both phases is added together whilst the AP as a negative potential is added to itself displayed as a positive potential and therefore approximates to zero (Fig. 4.23).

Isolation of SP. The SP obtained by ECochG is enhanced in certain pathological conditions such as Ménière's disorder. The SP, with few exceptions, occurs in a negative direction regardless of the phase of the stimulus.

The SP does not adapt even at very fast ISI. If a fast stimulus presentation rate is used (e.g. 150 per second), the AP is drastically reduced in amplitude whilst the SP is unaffected. At these fast stimulus presentation speeds the waveform contains a relatively large contribution from the SP. To discover the exact extent of the SP contribution, one may subtract the potential obtained at a fast stimulation rate (mainly SP) from the potential obtained at a slower rate (e.g. seven stimuli per second) which is AP and SP. The SP, being identical in both traces, is removed so that the potential remaining is the difference between the AP at the two speeds of stimulation (Fig. 4.24). This method does not yield a normal AP since at fast ISI the latency of the AP increases by a few tenths of a millisecond. The subtraction displays an AP slightly reduced in amplitude and diphasic in shape. Nevertheless, this is a clinically useful technique since one can quickly determine the extent to which the SP or a similar potential is altering the waveform of the AP in pathological conditions.

Clinical use of ECochG

The ECochG is used for two distinct clinical purposes. Firstly it provides a completely reliable indication of the cochlear output which is not affected by sedation or by masking problems. Secondly, it offers a unique insight into the physiology of the cochlea and may be used to learn more about the nature of particular causes of hearing dysfunction.

As a measure of auditory acuity

It must be stressed that ECochG only measures the threshold of the auditory mechanism at the level of the first order cochlear neurones. More central lesions can affect the hearing without affecting the ECochG (see Fig. 4.35). The vast majority of children with hearing losses suffer from peripheral disorders and the rarer central defects are usually suspected by the clinician following neurological examination. Certainly, if the ECochG reveals reduced cochlear function, the child must be suffering from a hearing loss.

Click stimuli evoke a whole nerve action potential (WNAP) from the entire length of the basilar membrane but the largest component of this response is derived from the basal coil. The threshold of the WNAP usually indicates the auditory acuity to within 10 dB of the mean level obtained by pure tone audiometry for frequencies between 2–8 kHz (Aran *et al.*, 1971).

The compound AP evoked by frequency specific stimuli gives an indication of the auditory threshold at the corresponding frequency and may be compared directly with the pure tone audiogram. It is fairly simple to make accurate measurements of the threshold at frequencies of 1–8 kHz but 500 Hz stimuli do not always evoke identifiable responses close to the psycho-acoustic threshold and a gap of 10–40 dB is common. No workers have yet succeeded in evoking consistent responses to stimuli of 250 Hz or less. The time required to determine threshold levels at 500 Hz, 1 kHz, 2 kHz, 4 kHz and 8 kHz for both ears is about 2 hours even using a relatively fast stimulus presentation rate (20 per second). Spoor (1974) has devised a 'fast method' of ECochG (Fig. 4.25) which may prove of particular value to those workers whose prime concern is the auditory evaluation of young children. He presented a train of six stimuli of different intensities and analysed the six potentials evoked by this stimulus train within a 62.5 ms analysis period.

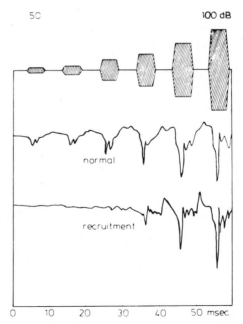

Fig. 4.25 The fast method of threshold electrocochleography achieved using a stimulus train of 4 kHz tone bursts. In the upper row, the stimulus series is shown schemmatically. The middle trace shows the action potentials in a normally-hearing ear. The lower trace shows the action potentials in an ear effected by a condition causing a recruiting hearing loss. (Odenthal, D.W., Eggermont, J.J. & Hermans, J. (1974), by permission *Revue de Laryngologie*).

In addition to threshold estimation, ECochG offers a sophisticated means of determing the nature of the hearing dysfunction and workers testing children can contribute further to the management of their patients by careful analysis of the data obtained. For instance, the slope of the amplitude/intensity function of the AP provides a good indication of recruitment, and a sharp rise in these functions suggests that a child may not tolerate a powerful hearing aid.

As an aid to neuro-otological diagnosis

The role of ECochG as a diagnostic tool is not yet as firmly established as its role in threshold prediction but it has certainly shown great promise in the diagnostic field. The topic is best discussed by considering the typical findings in various conditions.

The normal ear. The WN AP obtained from the normal ear shows a characteristic monophasic waveform at high stimulus intensity levels, the amplitude/intensity functions may be divided into 'H' and 'L' areas and the latency alters from approximately 1.2 ms at 110 dB HL to 4–6 ms at near threshold levels. These characteristics have been discussed fully earlier in this chapter.

The compound AP has an onset latency which progressively lengthens and a width which increases as the intensity of stimulation is reduced (*see* Fig. 4.9). Once the precise limits of the latency are known at different intensities (measured in dB SL), it is possible that a clinical application will be found.

The CM in the normal ear varies considerably but is usually of sufficient amplitude to be identifiable down to a level or pseudothreshold of approximately 60 dB SL. At intensities of 110 dB HL, the amplitude of the CM to click stimulation usually approaches the amplitude of the WN AP. The magnitude of the CM evoked by low frequency stimuli invariably exceeds that of the corresponding compound AP.

The SP in normal ears is usually identifiable as a small negative trough on the descending limb of the AP. This SP rarely affects more than one quarter of the length of the descending limb (Fig. 4.24). At low frequencies, such as 500 Hz, the SP contributes more to the AP and broadens the waveform; by using the subtraction technique to remove the SP, the 500 Hz AP is much more easily identified.

Conductive hearing losses. The ECochG obtained from a subject with a conductive hearing loss resembles the normal ECochG in practically every respect providing the same intensity of stimulation is being applied relative to the subject's hearing. The actual stimulus level in dB HL required to evoke the WN AP is greater in conductive deafness and so the amplitude/intensity and the latency/intensity functions when graphed show a 'shift to the right' similar to that seen in the speech audiogram. One may suspect a conductive hearing loss if the WN AP at 100 dB has a normal configuration but a latency of over 1.6 ms.

The CM in conductive pathologies is generally of a small amplitude despite the fact that the hair cells are unaffected. The explanation is simple; the CM at 110 dB HL in a case with a 40 dB conductive hearing loss is approximately equivalent to that of a normal ear at 70 dB HL. Similarly the SP is usually reduced in amplitude.

'Dead ears'.   A patient with no remaining cochlear function in one ear is occasionally misdiagnosed using subjective audiometric tests. The patient may be falsely suspected as having a severe conductive deafness since the sound applied to the skull near the damaged ear can travel to the unaffected, hearing ear. It is a surgical embarrassment to operate on a 'dead ear' expecting a conductive pathology, and it is a medico-legal embarrassment to operate on an only hearing ear unaware that if the operation fails the patient will be unable to hear from either ear. ECochG provides the only test of cochlear function in which no masking of the contralateral ear is required and provides a definite indication of residual cochlear activity.

Cochlear hearing losses.
   1. *Hair cell loss.*   Many cochlear pathologies result in damage to the hair cells. Recruitment has often been explained on the basis of selective damage to the outer hair cells.

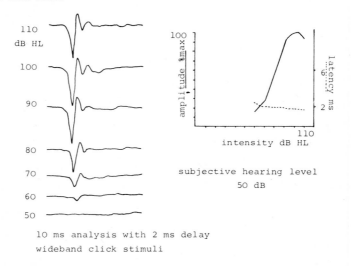

Fig. 4.26 The whole-nerve action potentials of a subject with a recruiting hearing loss and the corresponding input/output function. (Clear differences can be seen on comparing this figure with the normally-hearing subject in Fig. 4.12).

   Classically, such 'recruiting' hearing losses yield a diphasic WN AP (Fig. 4.26). This waveform is certainly not seen in every case of recruitment but when obtained it is virtually pathognomonic. The amplitude/intensity functions fall sharply to the threshold and the latency alters only slightly. These findings have been explained by Evans (1975a) as resulting from damage to the 'second filter' within the cochlea (*see* page 77). The amplitude/latency functions are much steeper than in normal ears as the latency at near threshold levels is shorter.
   The CM varies in amplitude but is generally smaller than normal. Rarely does the pseudo-threshold of the CM reach a lower level than the threshold of the AP except in severely deafened subjects. The SP is usually small.
   2. *High frequency hearing losses and acoustic trauma.*   In many cases in

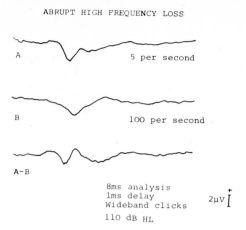

ABRUPT HIGH FREQUENCY LOSS

A   5 per second

B   100 per second

A—B

8ms analysis
1ms delay   2μV
Wideband clicks
110 dB HL

Fig. 4.27 The subtraction technique in a case of an abrupt high frequency hearing loss. The broadening of the waveform adapts and is shown to be of neural origin. (Gibson, W.P.R.& Beagley, H.A. (1976b), by permission *Revue de Laryngology*).

which the hair cell damage is confined almost entirely to the basal coil of the cochlea (e.g. acoustic trauma), the WN AP shows a characteristic late W waveform. The explanation lies with the observation that the waveform of the WN AP represents the neural activity from the entire length of the basilar membrane (Elberling, 1974). That part of the WN AP derived from the basal coil, which at high intensities is the N1, is reduced in amplitude whilst the later components of the WN AP derived from the middle coil of the cochlea are normal. The combined effect after suitable amplification results in the characteristic late W waveform. This waveform can be produced in normal subjects by introducing a high frequency masking noise with a low frequency cut off at 4 kHz. The late W is easily differentiated from broad AP waveforms seen in cases of Ménière's or eighth nerve tumours as the SP is small. Subtraction techniques (Fig. 4.27) do not alter the AP waveform to any great extent.

The CM in this condition is usually of minute amplitude presumably because all the outer hair cells close to the round window are affected.

3. *Sudden hearing loss.* A sudden hearing loss may result from many different causes ranging from profound anaemia to congenital syphilis, from multiple sclerosis to viral infection, from labyrinthine hydrops to vascular lesions of the brainstem and cochlea (Morrison and Booth, 1970). The electrocochleographic findings in these cases are as diverse as the multiplicity of aetiology would suggest. Iwata *et al.* (1976) have investigated many cases of sudden deafness. One of their most interesting findings was that those patients with relatively large negative SP contributions to the SP/AP complex had a significantly better prognosis than those patients with monophasic or diphasic waveforms. This finding would suggest that patients with labyrinthine hydrops fare better than those with other disorders, a finding which has been suspected clinically for some years. It is hoped that ECochG will prove useful in the differential diagnosis and management of sudden hearing losses.

4.   *Ototoxic cochlear damage*.   Aran and his colleagues (Aran, Darouzet and Erre, 1975) have noted specific changes in the WN AP in guinea pigs in the weeks following the administration of kanamycin. Several other studies have been performed in animals after the administration of either ototoxic antibiotics or other ototoxic agents but there has been little work concerning the electrophysiological changes which occur in man. There are, of course, many ethical problems which must be overcome before such a study is feasible. Recently, Ramsden, Wilson and Gibson (1977) have reported immediate effects occurring in the human cochlea after the infusion of the aminoglycoside tobramycin. Three subjects were studied on a total of five occasions whose clinical conditions required the urgent use of the drug. In every patient, to a variable extent, the WN AP altered within a few minutes of the drug administration and the change was most evident after approximately 1½ hours. The N1 component of the AP diminished and the N2 component became relatively more prominent so that the WN AP waveform resembled the form seen in cases with high frequency hearing losses (Fig. 4.28). In each case there was also a fall in the amplitude of the CM within a few minutes of drug administration. Usually these immediate changes were reversible. These studies in man gave similar results to those reported previously in the guinea pig by Brummett, Meikle and Vernon (1971). It appears that tobramycin affects predominantly the outer hair cells within the basal turn of the cochlea.

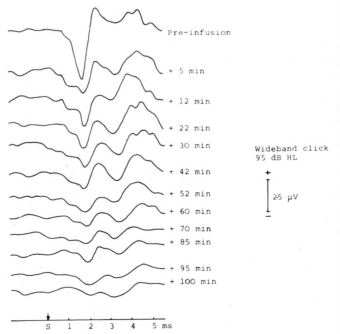

Fig. 4.28 The immediate electrocochleographic changes following intravenous infusion of tobramycin (Ramsden, R.T., Wilson, P. & Gibson, W.P.R. (1977), by permission *Annals of Otology, Rhinology and Laryngology*).

In a similar manner, electrocochleographic recordings have also been taken from patients receiving gentamicin (Ramsden, 1977). In no case was any change apparent during a two hour period after the infusion. Interestingly, a comparative study in the guinea pig has shown gentamicin to be more ototoxic than tobramycin (Brummett *et al.*, 1972). This illustrates the difficulty in determining the ototoxicity of a substance in man from animal experiments. ECochG may be of great value in offering an opportunity of assessing the early effects of a drug in the individual patient.

5. *Round window membrane rupture*. The author has tested two cases later shown at tympanotomy to be affected by rupture of the round window membrane. In each case the CM was virtually unobtainable and there was a slightly enhanced negative SP. The WN AP showed some recruitment in its functions and had a diphasic pattern. The finding that the CM was unobtainable would support the belief that the CM obtained by transtympanic electrocochleography is obtained only from hair cells situated on a limited area of the basilar membrane close to the round window membrane.

6. *Ménière's disorder*. It already appears that ECochG has a great deal to offer in the management and understanding of this disorder. Ménière's syndrome is characterised by a symptom triad of vertigo, hearing loss and tinnitus, and occurs commonly in many pathological conditions including vertebrobasilar insufficiency, congenital syphilis, auto-immune disorders, etc. Frequently, however, no underlying aetiology can be discovered and the condition, being idiopathic, is termed 'Ménière's disorder'.

Histological investigation has revealed an association between Ménière's disorder and distension of the endolymphatic compartment of the inner ear

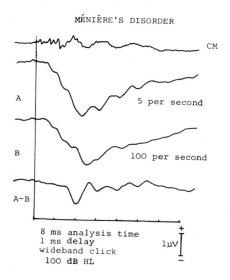

MÉNIÈRE'S DISORDER

Fig. 4.29 The subtraction technique in a case of Ménière's disorder. Note the relatively small CM and the relatively large SP component which is subtracted to reveal a small diphasic AP. (Gibson, W.P.R. & Beagley, H.A. (1976b), by permission *Revue de Laryngologie*).

(Hallpike and Cairns, 1938). Apart from the endolymphatic hydrops, the cochlea remains fairly normal histologically until the later stages of the disorder; the great majority of the hair cells appear intact and there is little evidence of retrograde degeneration of the nerve. The hearing fluctuates, especially in the lower frequency range, and it is postulated that this is a result of the endolymphatic hydrops which prevents the basilar membrane moving freely. The presence of loudness recruitment is probably related to a deterioration in the tuning curves of individual fibres similar, or identical, to the changes induced by cochlear ischaemia (see Fig. 4.3). The attacks of vertigo may either be related to dysfunction of the vestibular receptors due to anoxia or may be secondary to repeated rupture of Reissner's membrane with mixing of endolymph and perilymph (Lawrence and McCabe, 1959).

ECochG is valuable in the diagnosis and management of Ménière's disorder as it provides direct evidence of disturbed cochlear physiology; this is of especial value because there is no true animal model of the disorder. The commonest ECochG finding is a broadening of the SP/AP waveform, due entirely to a relative enhancement of the negative SP component (Fig. 4.29).

Schmidt, Eggermont and Odenthal (1974) have investigated the functions of the AP in Ménière's disorder. The amplitude/intensity changes are twice as steep in Ménière's disorder as in the normal cochlea. These changes indicate the presence of recruitment. The latency/intensity functions differ from those obtained in cases with hair cell loss; the span of latency is similar to normal, but abrupt transitions in the latency value around 55–65 dB only occur infrequently. Eggermont (1976), using the high pass masking technique described on page 78, has shown that the derived AP has a diphasic waveform.

Gibson, Moffat and Ramsden (1977) found that the more certain the clinical diagnosis of Ménière's disorder, the more likely there was to be widening of the SP/AP waveform. The presence of an abnormal SP may be related to the endolymphatic hydrops as Moffat (1977) has shown that the SP amplitude decreases after the administration of glycerol to the patient.

The CM in Ménière's disorder tends to be small and distorted. Gibson et al. (1977a) found that the CM evoked by a click stimulus at 110 dB HL was less than $2 \mu V$ peak to peak amplitude in 58 per cent of their series.

It appears that the presence of a broad SP/AP waveform and a small CM provides objective confirmation of the clinical diagnosis of Ménière's disorder. It is possible to use these abnormal responses as a means of monitoring the immediate effects of drugs. Gibson, Ramsden and Moffat (1977) infused a vasodilator (naftidrofuryl) intravenously. They found that whilst there was little change in the ECochG in normal cases, the abnormal responses often altered. The amplitude of the CM increased within a few minutes of the infusion and gradually, over several minutes, the amplitude of the negative SP decreased. These changes may provide evidence of a vascular aetiology in Ménière's disorder.

7. *Lermoyez's syndrome.* Lermoyez's syndrome is probably a variant of Ménière's disorder (Harrison and Naftalin, 1968). Schmidt and his colleagues (1975) have thoroughly investigated one case. Although the symptoms of vertigo

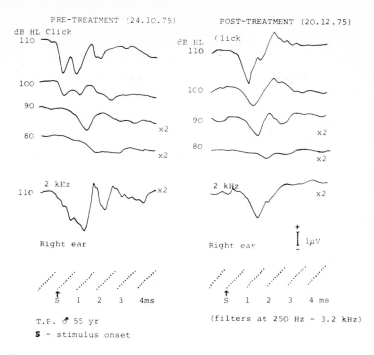

PRE-TREATMENT (24.10.75)   POST-TREATMENT (20.12.75)

Right ear

T.F. ♂ 55 yr

S - stimulus onset

(filters at 250 Hz – 3.2 kHz)

Fig. 4.30 The electrocochleogram obtained before and after penicillin and steroid therapy in a patient with congenital syphilis. (Ramsden, R.T., Moffat, D.A. & Gibson, W.P.R. (1977), by permission *Annals of Otology, Rhinology and Laryngology*).

and hearing impairment occur in the reverse sequence to Ménière's syndrome, the ECochG data for both conditions was similar. They noted the enhancement of the negative SP during hearing impaired periods and that the amplitude/latency functions lay within the normal limits.

8. *Syphilitic hearing loss.* In this condition, the endolymphatic hydrops is more marked than in Ménière's disorder and, in addition, there is extensive hair cell loss especially in the basal turn of the cochlea, with retrograde neural degeneration involving the spiral ganglion. Ramsden, Moffat and Gibson (1977) investigated a series of 30 ears mostly with the late onset congenital form of the disease. They reported that the CM was invariably minute. The AP was of small amplitude and often diphasic. In 77.7 per cent of cases, the SP affected more than one quarter of the descending (negative-going) limb of the AP (Fig. 4.30), but interestingly, the SP rarely affected the upgoing limb as it so commonly does in Ménière's disorder. Perhaps this finding is related to the difference in hair cell damage occurring in the two conditions.

9. *Tinnitus.* It is not possible to relate ECochG findings directly with tinnitus. The author has, nevertheless, encountered several young adults, aged 21–36 years, each suffering mainly from tinnitus; they complained also that their hearing was of poor quality even though pure tone audiometry failed to show any hearing loss. There was no vertigo. In each case the ECochG revealed a massive

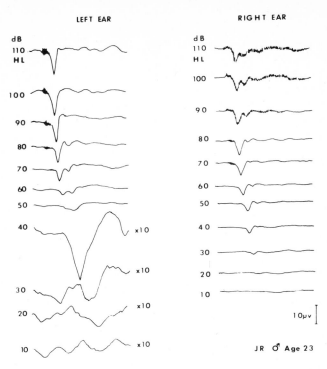

Fig. 4.31 The electrocochleogram of an ear affected by tinnitus. The hearing of both ears was normal. Note the massive CM in the affected ear.

CM in the affected ear which was superimposed upon the AP (Fig. 4.31) despite the use of stimulus phase alternation. The functional significance of this finding is unknown but one may surmise that some disorder has affected the cochlear efferent activity.

Retrocochlear hearing losses.

1. *Vestibulo-cochlear Schwannoma.*   A Schwannoma is a neoplasm arising from the Schwann cells of the myelin nerve sheath. In the case of the eighth cranial nerve, the origin is usually on the superior vestibular nerve. These are slow growing, benign tumours which eventually reach sufficient size to compress the brainstem and threaten the life of the patient (King, Gibson and Morrison, 1976). The early diagnosis of these tumours makes a great difference to the ease of surgical removal and to the mortality involved.

Morrison, Gibson and Beagley (1976) described a series of 67 ears with confirmed retrocochlear pathology (56 cases of Schwannoma). They proposed three criteria for reaching the diagnosis: broadening of the SP/AP waveform, observation of a large CM (over 5 μV peak to peak amplitude using a 110 dB HL click stimulus), and the presence of an AP at stimulus intensities less than the psychophysical threshold and inaudible to the patient. This last criterion was found to be the most certain but only occurred in one third of the patients, usually those with the larger, medially-placed tumours.

Odenthal and Eggermont (1976) have examined the derived AP using high pass masking in cases with eighth nerve tumours and report that the waveform is often monophasic. This is a most useful observation as it aids considerably in the differential ECochG diagnosis between Ménière's disorder (diphasic derived AP) and retrocochlear pathology (monophasic AP). The monophasic shape of the derived AP may be explained as a conduction defect in the passage of the nerve impulse (Beagley, *et al.,* 1977).

The broadening of the SP/AP waveform may be explained by the convolution of monophasic unit potentials. Recent work (Gibson and Beagley, 1976b) however, has suggested that the broadening is due to the superimposition upon the AP waveform of an SP-like potential (Fig. 4.32). A similar potential has been reported in the denervated cat cochlea by Kiang and Peake (1960) and named the slow component (SC). The SC does not adapt as readily as the AP and its onset latency differs from that of the SP (Gibson and Beagley, 1977). The SP/AP waveform was widened by over 4 ms in 71 per cent of the patients with tumours (Gibson and Beagley, 1976b).

In many of the patients with eighth nerve tumours, there is a brief positive wave preceding the broad negative SP/AP waveform. This wave probably represents a positive SP component which may be related to hair cell damage close to the round window membrane.

In the series of Gibson and Beagley (1976b), the CM in over 90 per cent of cases was large and could be compared with the amplitude of the CM in the unaffected ear. In some cases the CM appeared to be abnormally large. Admittedly the amplitude of the CM is extremely variable depending on electrode position and other factors, but the group findings are quite different from those in Ménière's disorder (Gibson and Beagley, 1976b).

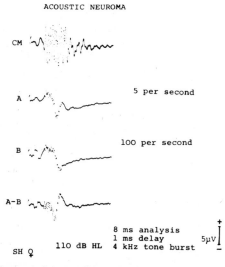

Fig. 4.32 The subtraction technique applied to the recordings from an ear affect by an acoustic neuroma (vestibulo-cochlear Schwannoma). (Gibson, W.P.R. & Beagley, H.A. (1976b), by permission *Revue de Laryngologie*).

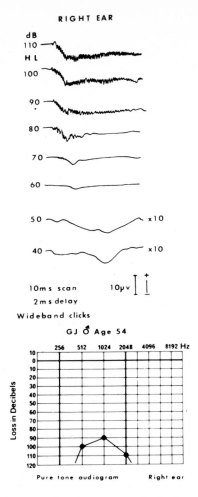

Fig. 4.33 The electrocochleogram obtained from a man with a brainstem astrocytoma affecting the hearing of the right ear (Beagley, H.A. & Gibson, W.P.R. (1976), by permission *Academic Press*).

2.   *Other pathologies affecting the eighth nerve.*   In general, any lesion affecting the eighth nerve affects the ECochG in the same manner as a Schwannoma (Beagley and Gibson, 1976). Intracochlear neurofibromatosis, a condition in which the tumour affects the nerve at the modiolus, usually results in a very wide SP/AP waveform. Basilar artery ectasia (Gibson and Wallace, 1975) does not produce much widening of the SP/AP waveform. The more medial the site of the pathology, the less likely it is to produce widening and the more likely it is that the objective ECochG threshold will be more sensitive than the psychophysical hearing threshold.

3.   *Brainstem lesions.*   Aran and his colleagues (1971) describe the ECochG in cases of kernicterus, a condition in which the basal ganglia of the brain are damaged by bile staining in the presence of high bilirubin levels in the blood. This

most commonly occurs in cases of haemolytic disease of the newborn which is due to rhesus incompatibility between the baby and its mother. Apart from lesions in the basal ganglia, there often is damage to brainstem nuclei, particularly the cochlear nuclei, resulting in deafness and other neurological defects. The ECochG, according to Aran *et al.* (1971) yields a broad SP/AP often with a sharp positive peak at its onset. They describe this waveform as 'anormale'.

Beagley and Gibson (1976) describe the ECochG results obtained from a man with a brainstem astrocytoma (Fig. 4.33). The findings are interesting because they illustrate in the one case all the criteria necessary for making the diagnosis of a retrocochlear lesion.

Lesions which affect the brainstem above the level of the cochlear nuclei may not affect the ECochG. Figure 4.34 shows an example. A young barrister had an 80 dB hearing loss in the left ear (confirmed by CERA) and yet provided a normal ECochG from that ear with an objective threshold of 20 dB. At surgery, a large vestibular Schwannoma was removed and it was noted that there was little evidence of damage to the vestibular or cochlear nerves actually within the internal acoustic meatus but that the tumour appeared to be pressing firmly into the brainstem. ECochG alone cannot differentiate between medially placed tumours and non-organic hearing loss, but if it is combined with another method of ERA, such as BER or CERA, the site of the lesion may be determined with certainty.

Final remarks

Although this chapter has dealt mainly with transtympanic ECochG, it is hoped that soon a less invasive method will be developed. At present, the use of a

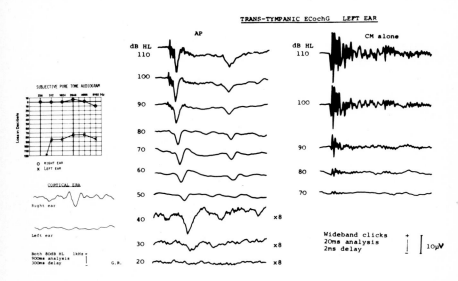

Fig. 4.34 The ECochG, CERA and PTA (pure tone audiogram) of a patient with a large eighth nerve tumour which arose medially from the left vestibular nerve and exerted its pressure mainly upon the brainstem (Morrison, A.W., Gibson, W.P.R. & Beagley, H.A. (1976), by permission *Clinical Otolaryngology*).

transtympanic electrode precludes experimentation and recordings can only be made when these are directly beneficial to the patient. The ECochG has a great deal to offer the otologist as it is a fundamental measure of peripheral auditory function which has promise in the diagnosis, understanding and treatment of sensorineural hearing loss.

5. The (Acoustic) Brainstem Electrical Responses—BER

BER represent probably the most exciting advance in ERA to date. Once certain remaining problems have been solved, such as the frequency specificity of the responses, it can be predicted confidently that BER will develop into a precise, valuable clinical tool. BER are obtained from surface electrodes by a completely safe and non-traumatic technique which may be performed by any sensible person without the necessity for medical training. The responses may be used as an objective means of assessing hearing acuity and are not affected by sedation. They may be also used for neuro-otological diagnosis.

The history of these responses really began in 1967 when Sohmer and Feinmesser, in Jerusalem, succeeded in recording the eighth nerve action potential (AP) from an active electrode placed on the earlobe. The magnitude of the AP was approximately $0.5\,\mu$V as evoked by a click of 115 dB SPL. For a few years their technique aroused little interest and more than a little scepticism regarding its clinical value. Then Jewett (1970) published his important work which confirmed the validity of the responses. Jewett and Williston (1971) showed that acoustically generated 'early' potentials could be detected from a wide area of the skull. Borrowing concepts and terminology from engineering they distinguished between two parts of a volume conducted field: the near field and the far field. Transtympanic electrocochleography is a near field technique in that the position of the active electrode is critical and repositioning it less than one centimetre further from the round window results in a loss of nine-tenths of the amplitude of the response. BER is a far field technique and the position of the active electrodes are not so crucial.

The finding which makes BER potentially such a valuable tool was that following the AP, responses were obtained which formed an interesting series of waves. Jewett (1970) postulated on the basis of cat recordings that there were four (vertex) positive waves following the AP which he related to specific generators within the brainstem. Lev and Sohmer (1972) performed similar work with cats and reached exactly the same conclusions except that they concentrated on the (vertex) negative waves. They concluded that the first wave arose from the first order cochlear fibres and was synonymous with the AP recorded by transtympanic electrocochleography, the second wave arose from the cochlear nucleus, the third wave arose from the superior olivary complex and the fourth and fifth waves arose from the inferior colliculus. Later Sohmer and Feinmesser (1973) demonstrated systematic variations in the response on changing the electrode positions in human subjects, these variations correlated well with the origins suggested by their earlier work. Buchwald and Huang (1975) have published the results of further investigations in cats. They found that the potentials were identified only after the kitten reached the age of two weeks and that the waveform seen in the adult cat was obtained at an age between one and two months. Their work suggested origins close to those previously suggested:

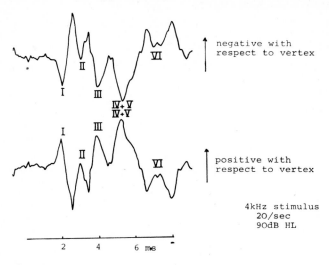

Fig. 5.1 A typical young adult BER waveform showing the labelling of the peaks according to Jewett's classification. The upper trace shows the response with vertex negative (mastoid positive) waves as an upwards deflection. The lower trace is in the opposite polarity.

Sohmer Classification		*Jewett Classification*
N1	The first order fibres of the acoustic nerve	NI
N2	The cochlear nucleus	NII
N3	The superior olivary nucleus with fibres crossing the midline	NIII
N4 (a & b)	The ventral nucleus of the lateral lemniscus and pre-olivary region with equal contributions from crossed and uncrossed fibres	NIV NV
N5	The inferior colliculus mainly activated by crossed projections	NVI

Starr and Achor (1977) doubt, however that the V wave is generated by the inferior colliculus and have suggested that the generator lies caudal to this site

An alternative possibility, other than a neural origin of the BER, was that the later waves were due to acoustic ringing within the cochlea. The argument against this view is based on the variability of the input/output functions of each of the waves and that the interval between each peak is irregular. Moore (1972) provided further circumstantial evidence when he showed that the later peaks were unaltered even in the presence of the same long duration white noise that was used as a stimulus to elicit the response. All in all, the evidence for a neural origin for each wave of the BER is strong and has been accepted by most workers. Thus BER have great neurological significance as they demonstrate the course of the auditory response through the important brainstem areas and, one hopes, reveal the site of any pathology which disrupts this passage.

Terminology

The terminology is at present confusing as it is yet to be standardised and different research groups are using different terms to describe the same events. Partly, this is due to the manner in which the subject evolved. Sohmer and Feinmesser (1967) named the response 'electrocochleography' as originally they were concerned with only the first wave (AP). Later, Jewett and Williston (1971) used the term 'auditory evoked far fields' to differentiate the response from near field techniques, but this term does not exclude the later cortical responses. Terkildsen and his group (1973) suggested 'far field electrocochleography', but in view of the importance of the latter parts of the response complex which are derived from brainstem structures, this term would seem inappropriate, as it implies that these responses only afford a measure of cochlear function. Hecox and Galambos (1974) used the term 'Brainstem auditory evoked responses' which seems a most apt description. The author has taken licence and altered this to 'Acoustic brainstem electrical responses' merely because the response can be obtained from a decerebrate animal in which the term 'auditory' seems inappropriate and because the International ERA study group (Davis, 1971) favour the term '*electric* response audiometry'. The argument is academic. The commonest abbreviation in recent literature is 'BER', as the word acoustic or auditory is ommitted.

The labelling of the various peaks has led to some confusion. There are six or more early mastoid negative peaks but the fourth and fifth are often merged together (Fig. 5.1). Some workers do not recognise the fourth and fifth waves as being truly separate—Sohmer and his colleagues label the peaks N4a and N4b respectively and the sixth wave as N5. Other workers such as Jewett designate the fourth, fifth and sixth waves as NIV, NV and NVI respectively. The reader has to take care, therefore, when reading the literature, to recognise the use of Roman numerals in Jewett's classification, for otherwise he may confuse N5 and NVI!

The FFP7, often mentioned in the literature, is the 'following–five peak' occuring at about 7 milliseconds after the stimulus onset. It is a particularly good area of the BER waveform for estimating threshold levels.

A final point: it is customary in electrophysiology to display negative peaks as up-going peaks. Some clinicians find it easier to recognise a down-going peak and in certain circumstances, such as transtympanic electrocochleography, it has become almost standard to display the waveform as obtained from the active electrode in the opposite polarity—with the negative peak displayed as a down-going peak. In BER, both the mastoid electrode and the vertex electrode are active so it is necessary to state the polarity with reference to one of the electrodes. In the illustrations shown in this chapter, the polarity is determined by the vertex electrode but many other workers provide illustrations in exactly the opposite mode. There is no definite rule yet regarding the manner in which the BER waveform should be displayed. The only vital requirement is that all the responses should be clearly labelled in Roman or Arabic numerals and that the polarity with respect to either the mastoid or vertex electrode must be specified.

The anatomy and neurophysiology of the central auditory pathway

An understanding of the central auditory pathway is needed to appreciate the significance of BER. A brief description follows but those interested in the subject are advised to consult the excellent monograph by Whitfield (1967). Most of the studies mentioned have involved animals such as the cat and some caution must be exercised in translating this work into the realm of human physiology. Kiang (1968) warns that there is considerable variation in the appearance of the various nuclei among different species as the pathway proceeds centrally. The pathway becomes more complex the higher the evolutionary status of the animal.

The acoustic nerve

The spiral ganglion contains the cell bodies of the first order neurones. The dendrites of these mainly bipolar sensory neurones terminate in functional contact with the hair cells of the organ of Corti. Their centripetal axons form the acoustic (cochlear) nerve which passes through the internal acoustic meatus to enter the brainstem in the groove between the pons and the medulla. In the acoustic nerve, the axons from the spiral ganglion are coiled along the nerve axis in the same direction as the cochlear turns (Lorente de Nó, 1933a; Sando, 1965).

The cochlear nuclei

Every fibre of the acoustic nerve ends by dividing in a regular manner to send a branch to the dorsal and ventral regions of the primary cochlear nuclei. These nuclei may be divided into thirteen different histological areas (Lorente de Nó, 1933b), or alternatively, the ventral nucleus can be divided into six regions on the basis of the outgoing fibres in the rat (Harrison and Irving, 1966). Despite this, most workers prefer simply to divide the nuclei into ventral and dorsal regions. Within these regions, the orderly tonotopographic organisation of the nerve is preserved, albeit in an altered form (Rose, Galambos and Hughes, 1959).

Every fibre not only makes contact with hundreds of cells in all regions of the nuclei, but since there are approximately twice as many cell bodies as acoustic nerve fibres, it follows that every cell body must make contact with hundreds of fibres. The cell bodies are also concerned with the efferent fibres described by Rasmussen (1942) and there are numerous inter-connecting fibres within the nuclei themselves.

No first order neurone passes beyond the primary cochlear nuclei (Kiang *et al*., 1965), although a small number of neurones do synapse within aberrant cell bodies within the acoustic nerve itself (Galambos and Davis, 1948). It is certain that the primary cochlear nuclei act as the first 'coding' and 'sorting' centre for auditory impulses. Inhibitory and excitatory functions are performed (Whitfield, 1967), helping to isolate the most important impulses and dispatch them to various other centres.

The functional importance of two parallel cochlear nuclei is not at all clear. They have separate efferent pathways but these merge again at higher levels. A major difference is that the entire output of the dorsal nucleus crosses the brainstem, by-passes the superior olivary complex and reaches the lateral lemniscus directly. The dorsal nucleus also sends fibres to the cerebellum and in many respects it seems as if it has retained features of a more primitive sensory system (Whitfield, 1967). The fibres of the ventral nucleus are distributed to the nuclei of the superior olivary complex on both sides of the brainstem, establishing the lowest level of binaural interaction.

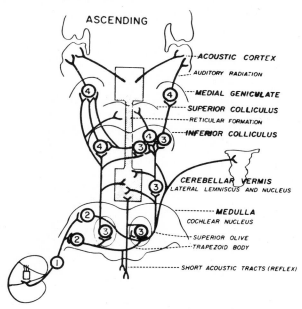

Fig. 5.2 A diagram of the afferent pathways of the eighth cranial (auditory) nerve.

The efferent 'outflow' of the cochlear nuclei

The main outflow of the cochlear nuclei is in a centripetal direction to make contact with other nuclei higher in the brainstem. The fibre diameter of this outflow consists of both the thickest and the thinnest seen in the ascending pathways of the CNS. Most of the fibres leave by coursing through the acoustic striae. The fibres in these striae follow four main projections (Fig. 5.2.):

1. From the rostral parts of the dorsal cochlear nucleus to the cerebellar auditory centres in the tuber vermis.

2. From the caudal parts of the dorsal cochlear nucleus to the contralateral lateral lemniscus and thence to the inferior colliculus.

3. From the dorsal parts of the ventral cochlear nucleus to the contralateral superior olivary complex.

4. From the ventral parts of the ventral cochlear nucleus to the homolateral superior olivary complex.

The superior olivary complex (Fig. 5.3)

This constitutes the second main relay station of the central auditory pathway and is believed to account for the third wave of the BER. If the nuclei of the lateral lemniscus are regarded as a rostral extension of the superior olivary complex, then it can be stated that all the fibres that leave the cochlear nuclei terminate in cell groups in the complex lying between the ponto-medullary junction and the midbrain. There is considerable variation between the size of the cell groups in different species. In man, the number of cells in the olivary and lemniscal groups is equally divided. In the cat, most of the cells lie in the olivary division and, since most of the research has been performed on this animal, caution should be exercised in translating the findings into terms of human physiology. The following description is based mainly on the reviews by Jungert (1958) and Whitfield (1967).

The superior olivary complex may be divided into at least six parts.

1. The lateral superior olive. This is a large S-shaped mass in the cat, but is poorly developed in man. The principal afferents come from the ipsilateral cochlear nucleus and the efferents are mainly distributed to the lateral lemniscus on both sides. Galambos, Schwartzkopff and Rupert (1959) have shown that the units in this nucleus cannot be driven by contralateral stimulation. The nucleus

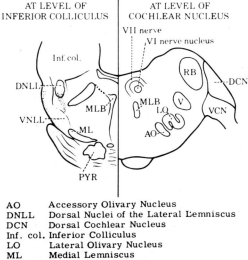

AO	Accessory Olivary Nucleus
DNLL	Dorsal Nuclei of the Lateral Lemniscus
DCN	Dorsal Cochlear Nucleus
Inf. col.	Inferior Colliculus
LO	Lateral Olivary Nucleus
ML	Medial Lemniscus
MLB	Medial Longitudinal Bundle
PYR	Pyramidal Tracts
RB	Restiform Body
V	Root of Vth nerve
VCN	Ventral Cochlear Nucleus
VNLL	Ventral Nuclei of the Lateral Lemniscus

Fig. 5.3 A cross-sectional diagram of the acoustic structures in the brainstem at the level of the cochlear nucleus and the inferior colliculus (Gibson (1974), by permission *London University*).

also sends efferents to the olivocochlear bundles and connects with the pre-olivary nuclei.

2.   *The medial superior olive (Accessory nucleus).*   This is not only the most fascinating nucleus in the superior olivary complex but also the largest of the nuclear masses in man. The afferents are derived from the cochlear nuclei of both sides. The nuclear cells have medially and laterally directed dendrites (Papez, 1930). The fibres from the contralateral ear end on the medially directed dendrites whilst those from the ipsilateral ear end on the laterally directed dendrites.

Galambos *et al.* (1959) found that, if an electrode was slowly advanced laterally through the nucleus, the polarity of the evoked response to contralateral clicks changed from negative to positive. The responses were almost mirror images and they found that, when both ears were stimulated simultaneously, there was almost complete cancellation of the response at the electrode tip.

Hall (1964) made a study of the responses in single neurones within the accessory nucleus. Most of the units were activated only by contralateral stimuli. An ipsilateral stimulus had no effect on its own but, when presented with a contralateral stimulus, it reduced the response to the latter. He also described some units that had the opposite effect and summed the response to the two stimuli. Furthermore, Moushegian, Rupert and Whitcomb (1964) have dis-covered a few units which are activated by ipsilateral stimuli and are inhibited by the coincident arrival of a contralateral stimulus.

The time/intensity trading effect of most units is as follows. If the click intensity is the same, then the response diminishes as the ipsilateral click is advanced in time relative to the contralateral click. If the timing is kept constant then the response increases as the ipsilateral click is made relatively less intense. If the contralateral click is 20 dB or more louder than the ipsilateral click, then the response becomes relatively independent of the timing of the two clicks. This remarkable sensitivity of the cells to the relative arrival of stimuli from the two ears within the time course of $\pm$ 500 microseconds and to relative stimulus intensities of 0–20 dB corresponds to the ranges of time and intensity as a sound source is moved around the head. One may postulate that this nucleus is concerned especially with the processing of directional information.

A further remarkable finding is that the onset latency of the evoked response is in the order of 5–10 milliseconds (Galambos *et al.*, 1959; Hall, 1964). This is much later than one would calculate from the number of synapses that the response is known to have bridged and most surprising when it can be shown that the first cortical responses in the same cat have a latency of only 12 milliseconds. Galambos *et al.* (1959) commented on the consistency of this timing during repeated trials in the same animal using the same stimulus parameters. The majority of efferent fibres pass to the medial portions of the lateral lemniscus on both sides. There are also connections to motor nuclei including the facial nerve.

3.   *The medial and lateral pre-olivary nuclei.*   Stotler (1953) stated that the afferent fibres come entirely from the ipsilateral cochlear nucleus and most of the efferent fibres pass to the ipsilateral lateral lemniscus. There are, also, collaterals between the pre-olivary nuclei and the other superior olivary nuclei, in particu-

lar connecting with the accessory nucleus and the lateral 'S-shaped' nucleus.

4.   *The nuclei of the trapezoid body*.   Stotler (1953) believed that the afferent fibres came entirely from the contralateral cochlear nucleus but Lewy and Kobrak (1936) suggested that there were also ipsilateral afferents. The efferent connections are not known with certainty, although Rasmussen (1946) on the basis of degeneration studies in cats believed that some fibres descended in the medial longitudinal bundle and tectospinal tract to make contact with motor nuclei.

5.   *The nuclei of the lateral lemniscus*.   These may be divided into a ventral nucleus which forms an extension of the lateral pre-olivary nucleus (suggested as the source of the fourth wave of BER by Buchwald and Huang, 1975) and a dorsal or commisural nucleus which follows a circumscribed line along the entire length of the lateral lemniscus. The nuclei receive second order fibres from the contralateral dorsal cochlear nucleus and Jungert (1958) has demonstrated a few ipsilateral second order fibres from the ventral cochlear nucleus. The vast majority, however, of the efferents from the ventral cochlear nucleus synapse within the superior olivary complex before reaching the lateral lemniscus on both sides. ·

The efferent fibres pass mainly to the ipsilateral inferior colliculus. Jungert (1958) has shown that the fibres which cross never recross and, if a transverse hemisection is made of the ipsilateral brainstem above the level of the superior olivary complex, all ipsilateral collicular responses are abolished. Some fibres, also, establish contact with cells of the reticular system and others with tracts leading to motor nuclei. Rasmussen (1960) has shown that centrifugal efferents arise from the nuclei of the lateral lemniscus and travel back to the dorsal cochlear nucleus.

6.   *The retro-olivary cell group*.   The origin of the afferent fibres to this nucleus remains uncertain. Rasmussen (1946, 1960) has shown that it provides efferents to the crossed olivo-cochlear bundle. The outgoing fibres cross the midline just below the VIth nucleus to be joined by uncrossed fibres from the lateral 'S-shaped' olivary nucleus.

The cerebellar connections

There appears to be considerable connection between the auditory system and the lobulus simplex and tuber vermis regions of the cerebellum. Snider and Stowell (1944) found that the cerebellar responses were abolished on destruction of the inferior colliculus but not on higher decerebration. They have shown, however, that stimulation of the temporal lobe produces responses in the cerebellum. Only the pathway from the dorsal cochlear nucleus to the auditory cerebellum has been demonstrated histologically at present (Niemer and Cheng, 1949) and the other more complex connections await anatomical recognition.

The lateral lemniscus

The lateral lemniscus is a short tract that delivers at least third order fibres from the cochlea on both sides to the inferior colliculus. A tonotopographic representation is maintained. Considering the frequency distribution in the inferior colliculus, it is likely that the most medial portion carries the highest frequency information and the frequency distribution changes gradually until the lowest frequencies are carried in the most laterally placed fibres.

The inferior colliculus

Cajal (1909) believed that the inferior colliculus was concerned only with reflex activities whilst the fibres bound for the cortex by-passed the structure entirely. Barnes, Magoun and Ranson (1943) were the first to demonstrate that this belief was erroneous and that, in the monkey, the vast majority of fibres relayed in the inferior colliculus. Histologically it consists of five layers. It is the highest level at which fibres cross from the auditory pathway on one side to the other (Ades and Brookhard, 1950). Rose *et al.* (1963) have demonstrated an orderly tonotopographical distribution across the collicle. Erulkar (1959) has shown that certain neurones are excited by a stimulus to one ear and modified by a simultaneous stimulus to the other. Most commonly, the responses to bilateral stimuli are summed. He also showed that if the first stimulus preceded the second by more than four milliseconds, then the response to the latter was entirely suppressed. If the source of the stimulus was moved around the head from the contralateral to the ipsilateral side, the onset latency lengthened. It would be fascinating to repeat this experiment with BER as it appears that the inferior colliculus has some role in processing the data concerned with localisation.

In addition to its function as a relay station, it is known that the central grey matter of the inferior colliculus contains minor reflex connections in man. Incidentally, in bats the inferior colliculus is enormous.

The superior colliculus

The superior colliculus is mainly concerned with the visual reflex pathways. There are, however, some auditory fibres which pass from the lateral lemniscus to the structure and it may be that visual and auditory activities are co-ordinated here (Davis, 1951). It is, perhaps, the route of the response in auditory electro-oculomotography (Utsumi, Inui and Inui, 1966), a method of objective audiometry not reviewed in this book but mentioned in discussion of CNV (Chapter Seven).

The medial geniculate body

The medial geniculate body is functionally part of the thalamus. It consists of a small celled pars principalis and a large celled par magnocellaris (Rioch, 1929). Morest (1964) has recognised further smaller nuclei. The majority of fibres are at least fourth order neurones, although a few third order neurones may reach the structure direct. The pars principalis appears to be the only part concerned with the auditory pathway (Rose and Woolsley, 1949). A weak tonotopicity has been demonstrated by Purser and Whitfield (1972) and Rubel and Parks (1975). Its main output is to the primary cortical areas and, perhaps, to the centrifugal pathway. Chang (1960) demonstrated the presence of electrical circuits which reverberate between the medial geniculate body and the auditory cortex.

The auditory cortex

The boundaries of the auditory cortex are virtually impossible to determine either anatomically or functionally. Those parts of the cortex that receive and send fibres directly to and from the lower auditory centres are by definition 'primary auditory areas'. Secondary areas are connected to primary areas and, in turn, tertiary areas connect with secondary areas, and so on. Kiang (1955) and Downman, Woolsey and Lende (1960) have shown that not all the activation of secondary areas takes place via the primary areas. To confuse matters even more, it has been shown that primary areas may act as secondary areas at the same time. It is tempting to postulate that, as the response spreads to these more diffuse areas, functions linked with word recognition, speech, memory, etc. are served.

It is generally accepted that in man part of the primary auditory area lies in the superior temporal gyrus and that this extends into the transverse temporal gyri, lying in the floor of the posterior ramus of the lateral sulcus behind the insula. It is a matter of dispute whether the insula and other temporal gyri are primary or secondary areas. The extent of the secondary areas is not known but it seems likely that areas of the parietal and frontal lobes are involved.

The first cortical responses recorded directly from the exposed cortex in man occur with an onset latency of 10–30 milliseconds (Sem-Jacobsen et al., 1956; Chatrian, Petersen and Lazarte, 1960; Celesia et al., 1968). The early responses recorded by Mendel and Goldstein (1969) from the scalp may be identical (see Chapter Eight)

Some characteristics of the response

Electrode positions

The optimum electrode positions are not known yet with certainty but, since BER is a far field technique, small differences in electrode sites are not critical. Sohmer and Feinmesser (1973) have demonstrated the variations of the response obtained from different sites in human subjects. Most workers use bipolar electrode techniques with one electrode placed at the vertex and the other placed either over or near the ipsilateral mastoid process. Sohmer and Feinmesser (1973) use a clip electrode attached to the earlobe as this avoids some of the larger muscle potentials. Hecox and Galambos (1974), Thornton (1975a) and Suzuki (1975) place an electrode actually over the mastoid process and Terkildsen (1975) advises positioning the electrode on the neck a few inches behind the ipsilateral mastoid process. Placing an electrode on the vertex is not necessary as Davis and Hirsch (1977) have positioned the active electrodes over the mastoid process and on the forehead, immediately below the hairline with the earth electrode placed on the chin. Despite these differences in positioning one of the electrodes, the waveform of the BER remains basically unaltered.

Ipsilateral and contralateral responses

Terkildsen and his group (1973) showed the variation of the response to a unilateral stimulus according to whether it was recorded from the ipsilateral or contralateral mastoid. Figure 5.4 shows similar recordings obtained by the author. The BER waveform obtained from the ipsilateral mastoid (to vertex) shows the familiar profile, and the recording from the contralateral mastoid is in many respects similar except that NI is absent. Thornton (1975b) reported this matter at length and drew attention to his finding that the first negative peak on

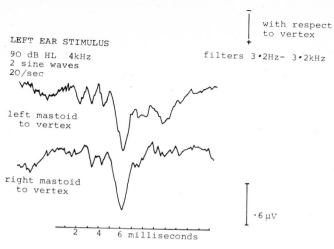

LEFT EAR STIMULUS

90 dB HL   4kHz
2 sine waves
20/sec

with respect
to vertex

filters 3·2Hz- 3·2kHz

left mastoid
to vertex

right mastoid
to vertex

·6 μV

2   4   6 milliseconds

Fig. 5.4 The ipsilateral BER (upper trace) and the contralateral BER (lower trace) from the same normally-hearing young adult subject.

the contralateral recording which is equivalent to the NII is often large. He discussed the possible explanations for the waveforms encountered, in a later article (Thornton 1976b). In general, the findings are compatible with the belief that the NI is derived from the first order cochlear nerve fibres and is the same potential as recorded by transtympanic electrocochleography, and the NII originates from the cochlear nucleus.

The absence of the NI in BER when using high stimulus intensities must always raise the suspicion that the stimulus is being delivered to a deaf ear in a subject with a unilateral hearing loss. The true situation is soon revealed if masking of the opposite ear is properly accomplished.

It is also likely that analysis of the ipsilateral and contralateral recordings will provide useful neurological information (Thornton and Hawkes, 1976a). The author has found that differences of over 1 millisecond between the NV of the two recordings only occurs in subjects with normal hearing when pathology, such as demyelination, is present.

Amplitudes of the BER

The BER are minute and the peak to peak amplitude of individual waves rarely exceeds 1 μv. With increasing stimulus intensity, the amplitude of the first wave increases in a similar manner to the action potential of transtympanic electrocochleography, except that it is some twenty times smaller. In a normal subject, it is usually possible just to identify the 'plateau' between the 'H' and 'L' areas of the graph. The amplitude of the later waves from the brainstem nuclei increases little with increasing stimulus intensity and at high intensities the amplitude occasionally is decreased.

The first wave, N1, is not usually identifiable using stimulus intensities of less than 25 dB SL (Thornton, 1975a). The second wave, N2, has the smallest amplitude of all the BER and can rarely be identified at low stimulus intensities.

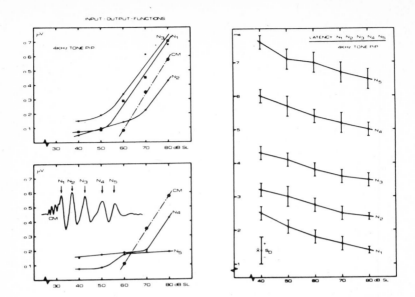

Fig. 5.5   The amplitude/intensity functions (left) and the latency/intensity functions of the BER. The filter bandpass was 0.5–4.5 kHz (24 dB/octave 'roll-off'). The intensity is recorded as dB SL. The latency values are based on the difference between the calculated arrival of the stimulus at the tympanic membrane and the maximum negativity for each peak. (Terkildsen, K., Osterhammel, P. & Huis In't Veld, F. (1973), by permission *Scandanavian Audiology*).

At the faster stimulus repetition rates (over 50 per second), the fifth wave, N4b or NV, is the largest in amplitude and it is this wave that can be seen most easily at stimulus levels close to the subject's psychophysical threshold.

The amplitude/intensity functions of BER at a stimulus presentation rate of 10 per second are shown in Figure 5.5 (Terkildsen, Osterhammel and Huis In't Veld, 1973). (It must be remembered that Terkildsen and his group use Sohmer's classification of N1–N5, and a high pass filter at 500 Hz with a sharp slope (24 dB/octave) which attenuates N4 and N5).

Latencies of the BER

The latency of each of the BER peaks, using the similar stimuli, is remarkably constant amongst adult subjects. The latency of each of the waves decreases by almost similar amounts as the stimulus intensity increases. The NV wave almost invariably follows NI after 4 ms exactly. Figure 5.5 also shows the intensity/latency functions of each of the BER peaks and also indicates the statistical probability of the response occurring at a given point (Terkildsen *et al.*, 1973). With increasing stimulus presentation rates, there is no alteration of the latency of NI but the latency of the later waves does increase slightly (Pratt and Sohmer, 1975), the latency change of each wave being greater than that of the waves preceding it (accumulative effect).

The latencies of the BER are prolonged in neonates (Hecox, 1975). The NV (N4b) in a one day old baby has a latency of approximately 7.6–8.6 milliseconds at 60 dB SL.

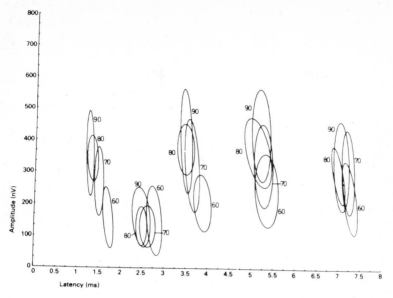

Fig. 5.6 Bivariate probable ellipses of amplitude by latency for the responses N1–N5. Intensity as dB SL. Bandpass 100 Hz to 4 kHz. (Thornton, A.R.D. (1975b), by permission *Scandanavian Audiology*).

Latency/amplitude probabilities

Thornton (1974, 1976a) has analysed the BER responses from six normal subjects and has calculated statistical limits for normal amplitude and latency functions at different stimulus levels (Fig. 5.6).

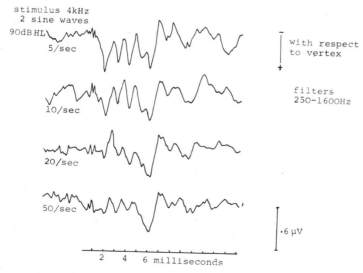

Fig. 5.7 The alteration of the BER waveform resulting from different rates of stimulus presentation.

Effect of binaural stimulation

Blegvad (1976) has shown that if the stimulus is delivered to both ears simultaneously, then binaural summation occurs. A 50 dB binaural stimulus evokes an equal amplitude to that of an 80 dB monaural stimulus. The implications during free-field testing are evident.

Effect of prolonged or repeated stimulation (habituation)

The amplitude and latency functions of BER are remarkable constant on repeated or prolonged stimulation. Thornton (1974) and Thornton and Coleman (1975) found no significant variations in six normally hearing subjects who had four replicates of four stimulus levels during two test sessions.

Effect of stimulus presentation rate (equilibration)

The N1 response diminishes with shorter interstimulus intervals. In effect, it begins to decrease at stimulus presentation rates of 10 per second and it is difficult to identify in BER at rates over 50 per second. The amplitude of the later

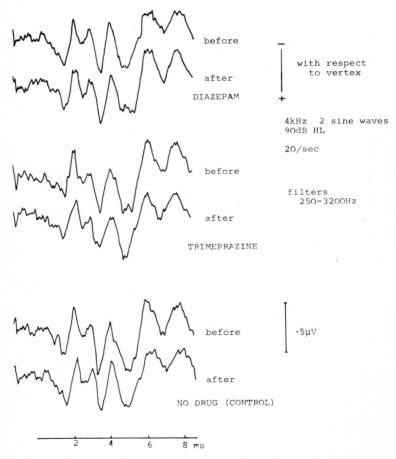

Fig. 5.8 The effect of two sedatives (diazepam and trimeprazine) upon the BER waveform.

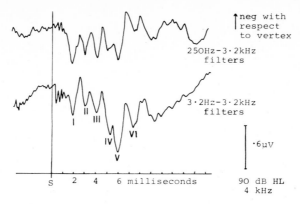

Fig. 5.9 The alteration of the BER waveform resulting from altering the bandwidth of the recording apparatus. Upper trace: 250 Hz to 3.2 kHz. Lower trace: 3.2 Hz to 3.2 kHz.

waves, however, appears to be little affected even at the faster rates of 50–100 per second (Pratt and Sohmer, 1975; Terkildsen, Osterhammel and Huis In't Veld, 1976), but the author notes that NIV and NV tend to merge at faster rates. This property of the later waves is useful as it allows the collection of a large number of epochs within a reasonable period when threshold estimations are being sought. Figure 5.7 shows the effect on the BER waveform of varying the stimulus presentation rate.

Effect of sedation

The BER do not appear to be affected by sedatives, or even by general anaesthetic agents and relaxants. Bryant (1976) investigated the effects of two different sedatives in six normal subjects. After administering diazepam and trimeprazine, he found no significant alterations of the BER waveforms (Fig. 5.8). This is a considerable advantage in testing young children; the author always tests young children whilst they are asleep and has found no difficulty in obtaining clear responses.

The bandwidth of BER

Fourier analysis of the BER shows that most of their energy lies in the range of 800–1200 Hz. The use of narrow bandwidth filtering does lead to some distortion of the responses. The N1 response in certain circumstances contains low frequencies (Chapter Four) so, if a high, high pass filter (over 100 Hz) is used, the N1 response will not show the same characteristic waveforms as the transtympanic AP. The cochlear microphonic, also, contains energy at low frequencies and is most clearly seen with wide bandwidth filter settings. The later responses are even more distorted by high, high pass filtering and the NV wave only reaches 70 per cent of its true amplitude when a 250 Hz filter is employed (Terkildsen *et al.*, 1976). The baseline of the response complex is more curved, accentuating the later waves when wide filter limits are used. If a 250 Hz high pass filter is introduced, the response baseline becomes almost flat (Fig. 5.9).

The advantage of employing a high, high pass filter is that low frequency artefacts which may disrupt the response, making identification of the peaks hazardous, are excluded. The filters used by various clinical groups vary between 100–500 Hz (high pass) to 3–5 kHz (low pass). The effectiveness of the filters depends, greatly, on the sharpness of their cut-off frequencies.

In conclusion, it is evident that one cannot compare the waveforms obtained by different workers directly unless the rate of stimulus presentation, the polarity of the recordings and the filter bandwidths (together with the slope of the filters) are known.

The frequency specificity of BER

It is difficult to identify BER unless there is good synchronisation of neural activity. BER suffer from the same problems as transtympanic electrocochleography when low frequency stimuli are employed (*see* detailed discussion in Chapter Four). Most workers agree that frequency specific responses may be obtained using tone bursts of 2 kHz or higher. Davis and Hirsh (1975) evaluated the use of a 500 Hz tone pip with a rise and fall of 2–3 ms, and found the NV wave at 30 dB SL was low in amplitude, rounded in waveform and had a latency of 10 ms. Above 40 dB SL, this response was obscured by a larger, earlier response. Nevertheless, further work (Davis and Hirsch (1977) has shown that BER can be used to estimate thresholds at 500Hz although the response threshold is at least 15dB above the behavioural threshold.

Another possible method of increasing the frequency range of BER is the use of high pass masking techniques (see Chapter Four) (Parker, 1976). Using these techniques Eggermont and Don (1977) have reported that the V wave is dominant using a 500Hz stimulus and shows excellent frequency specificity.

Frequency selective masking of tonal stimuli

Terkildsen, Osterhammel and Huis In't Veld (1975) have performed a series of selective masking experiments. They noted marked changes in the recordings when masking noise was centred at or above the frequency of the stimulus: the NV wave showed a shift in latency and the following peak was enhanced. The explanation is probably similar to that given by Elberling (1973), *see* Figure 4.10.

The test and test/retest reliability

The test reliability of BER is excellent. The NV peak can be used confidently to estimate the hearing status. The latency of this peak is remarkably constant even from subject to subject and, in normally-hearing adults, it occurs at 4.9–5.5 ms using an 80 dB HL click stimulus. The NV peak nearly always follows the NI peak by exactly 4.0 ms unless the subject has a disorder affecting the brainstem. For audiometric purposes, the NV can usually be identified at 10 dB SL or less using click stimuli or tone bursts of 2–8 kHz (Davis, 1976b). The exact percentage of subjects who do not yield an identifiable NV within 10 dB of their psychoacoustic threshold does not appear to have been reported but the author can state that he has never tested a subject who did not show the response at 30 dB SL using a 4 kHz stimulus; the older subjects, over 40 years of age, seemed the most difficult to test for threshold purposes. At lower stimulus frequencies, the NV becomes broader and more difficult to identify (Davis and Hirsch, 1976). Antonelli (1976), using a 1 kHz stimulus, reported that the BER threshold was between 10 and 30 dB for 75 per cent of his 39 adult subjects. At 500 Hz, the NV is very difficult to identify and Davis and Hirsch (1977) found difficulty in detecting the response within 15dB of the psychoacoustic threshold.

The rest/retest reliability is good. The BER waveform does not show any change on repeated or prolonged testing and Thornton and Coleman (1975) were unable to demonstrate any significant variation on repeatedly testing four normal subjects. Moreover, the BER waveform does not vary significantly on testing the same subject at separate sessions. Thornton (1975b) tested the same six subjects using the same stimuli on two different occasions and found no significant changes in either the amplitude or the latency of the BER. The standard deviations of the amplitude data were proportionally much larger than those obtained from the latency data. 'This suggests that despite the averaging procedure, a considerable proportion of the measured response amplitude variance is attributable to the remaining variance of the background noise process.' (Thornton, 1975b).

In conclusion, it appears that BER rivals ECochG in respect of test and test/retest reliability. The accuracy with which it may be used to estimate the hearing threshold even in the sedated child must make this response highly attractive to many ERA workers.

Instrumentation

Basically the apparatus is similar to that used in obtaining other ERA responses which has been described in Chapter 2. There are some special requirements for BER which will be listed. In general, these requirements are made necessary by the extremely small voltages of the response which rarely exceeds 1μ V in amplitude.

The test environment

The subject is best tested in a relaxed position which will minimise any myogenic activity, particularly that of the neck muscles, which may generate electrical artefacts. Most workers ask the subject to relax on a couch with a pillow placed under the neck to encourage the neck muscles to relax. Active children must be sedated (babies can be tested during natural sleep after feeds). Often testing is performed in a darkened room.

The stimulus generation

Stimulus requirements.   BER can only be satisfactorily obtained at present by using a very brief stimulus with sharp onset characteristics. At present clicks, filtered clicks and tone bursts are being used to obtain BER. A critical evaluation of each of these types of stimulus is given in Chapter Two.

Stimulus repetition rate.   Due to the minute voltages involved, many individual BER epochs have to be summed and averaged before the responses can be clearly identified from the background fluctuations.

Some subjects, typically young children and babies, only yield small BER and when intensities are used that are only slightly above the psychophysical hearing threshold, up to 8000 stimulations may be required to obtain an identifiable response. Most workers try to minimise the time taken to obtain each BER by using a fast stimulus repetition rate. Fortunately, the last two negative peaks, which give the best threshold measure, may be identified even at very fast interstimulus intervals. It is permissible to use a stimulus repetition rate of 50 per second and at this speed it takes 2 minutes and 40 seconds to record the BER to 8000 stimulus presentations. This is compatible with the bounds of clinical reality. The problem of using stimulus rates in excess of 50 per second is that myogenic responses, such as the post-aural response, become superimposed on the recordings, making interpretation hazardous.

When BER is to be employed as a neuro-otological tool, it is essential to obtain all the various peaks. Unfortunately, the earlier peaks do suffer if the stimulus presentation rate is increased, so for this kind of work a rate of 10 per second is advised. Generally intensities are used well above the subject's hearing threshold, allowing the responses to be obtained after 2000 stimuli. At this rate it takes 3 minutes and 20 seconds to obtain each BER recording.

Stimulus transducer.   When obtaining BER, care must be taken over the choice of the stimulus transducer. If a magnetic device is used without shielding, it will, when energised, be surrounded by a strong magnetic field. This field will produce artefacts which, when summed by the 'computer', obscure the BER. Care has to be taken to shield the transducer with 'mu-metal' which reduces the magnetic field.

If a loudspeaker is used (Thornton, 1975a), an anechoic test chamber is essential. Otherwise reverberations around the room will evoke secondary responses that will superimpose on the recording, making the interpretation hazardous. Most workers prefer magnetically-shielded headphones, which give good results. There can be some difficulties in fitting these to young children and babies unless they are heavily sedated. Terkildsen *et al*. (1973) use a hearing aid earphone (Beyer DT 507S, 10Ω) which is enclosed in a box with double wall of 'mu-metal'. The sound from this transducer is passed along an acoustically damped piece of plastic tubing which is fitted in an air-tight manner into the external acoustic meatus. This method has the advantage of producing a closed acoustic system.

Stimulus calibration.   Without wishing to be repetitious, a plea for care in calibrating the exact stimulus intensities at the tympanic membrane is made. Calibration in 5 dB steps is adequate, although some workers prefer the flexibility of 1 dB steps. Most workers use a physiological calibration for the transient stimuli and once this calibration is made, a physical means of maintaining the accuracy on a day to day basis. Details are given in Chapter Two.

Masking (random) noise.   The apparatus must include provision for the application of masking noise to the non-test ear if monaural information is sought. Clicks contain a wide spectrum of frequencies so wide band masking is required. Tone bursts or pips can be masked by narrow band masking. Fascinating neurological work may be done to show the effects of 'cross masking' on the various brainstem responses. High and low pass masking has also been used to increase the frequency selectivity of BER.

The recording equipment
The electrodes.   Surface electrodes are needed which are placed onto the

scalp and mastoid or neck of the subject. Any high quality EEG electrodes may be used. It is obviously an advantage to obtain the best possible contact between electrode and skin. The electrode impedance should ideally be 2.5 kΩ or less. Higher electrode impedance increases the noise to signal ratio and makes identification of these small potentials hazardous.

Amplifiers.   Low noise biological amplifiers are essential. The total gain must be at least 10^5 and preferably 10^6. The usual arrangement is to place one (pre-) amplifier close to the subject with a fixed gain of 10^3 and then to use a further (main) amplifier, situated close to the averager and display, to adjust the final gain of the signal.

Filter settings.   The high pass filter is commonly set at 100–500 Hz, which helps exclude low frequencies which may contain artefacts, for example, 50 Hz mains interference. If the cochlear microphonics are sought, a lower level for the high pass filter may be required. The low pass filter is usually set at 3 kilohertz to exclude high frequencies which may cause blurring of the traces.

The averager.   Any properly programmed computer can be used to record BER. Small purpose-built averagers (such as the Medelec DAV6) are adequate. The analysis period required varies from 20 milliseconds for young babies to 10 milliseconds for the majority of adult work. There should be a minimum of 10 memory addresses per millisecond so that the details of the responses may be properly resolved.

The monitor oscilloscope.   It is essential to be able to monitor the on-going unaveraged signal during the period in which each response is obtained. This on-going record is mainly a mixture of EEG signals and myogenic activity. Once experience has been gained, it becomes quite simple to detect abnormalities and sudden changes of this signal which may lead to artefacts contaminating the averaged response. It is also an advantage to be able to watch the averaged response building. For these purposes a two channel oscilloscope meets the minimum requirements.

Artefact rejection facilities.   Since the responses are small, it is wise to have artefact rejection facilities available. Each response may take as long as five minutes to obtain, so it can be very frustrating if it is suddenly obscured by a movement artefact close to completion.

Permanent recording of results.   Permanent records are useful for further analysis of the results after the test session. Any of the methods outlined in Chapter Two may be usefully employed.

Timing and amplitude calibration pulses should be included in each permanent recording.

Testing procedures

The procedure varies according to whether the subject is a cooperative adult or a young child or baby.

Co-operative subjects.   Adults and older children generally pose few problems during recording sessions. They should be tested whilst resting on a bed with a pillow placed under the neck to relax the neck musculature. Earphones are placed over the head.

The biological signal obtained from the patient may be examined by asking the patient to smile or grit his teeth; this manoeuvre should cause the signal noise to increase. Once the patient's signal has been seen to be satisfactory, the patient is asked to relax and sleep if possible. It is best to start BER procedures by eliciting the responses to a loud stimulus (e.g. 80 dB HL) so that the profile of the BER can be obtained clearly. The stimulus intensity is then reduced in regular steps which causes the BER to diminish, they can be identified by comparing them with the previous recordings. As the stimulus intensity becomes quieter, most subjects grow bored and may even sleep, and this reduces noise and allows clear recordings to be made at levels near threshold.

Young children.   Young children are difficult to test satisfactorily without the use of sedatives. Difficulties are often encountered on attempting to attach the electrodes and whilst reducing the impedance between the electrode and the skin to a satisfactory level. Undoubtedly, an experienced person can succeed in the majority of cases but not all clinics have such a person available. The second problem is that young children find it difficult to relax and may even grow bored or begin actively to resist testing. Fortunately, BER are not affected by sedatives or general anaesthesia. Burian (1975) summarised the use of different sedatives and found that the majority of clinics favoured the use of either promethazine (Phenergan®), trimeprazine (Vallergan®) or chlorpromazine (Largactil®). Spillman, Erdmann and Leitner (1975) report the use of alphadione (Althesin®) specifically during BER audiometry with good results. General anaesthesia rather than sedation may be employed but, if such a measure is necessary, surely

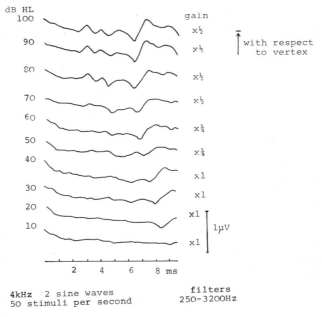

Fig. 5.10 The BER of a normally-hearing young adult. The NV is just identifiable at 10 dB HL (psychoacoustic threshold 5 dB HL)

the comparatively minor addition of a transtympanic electrode is reasonable, as the threshold level is more consistent and easier to identify with certainty.

Babies.   BER is an excellent means of assessing hearing acuity in babies, especially as it is a non-invasive technique. Often babies can be tested simply and without fuss after feeds but sometimes they will cry or move incessantly. The author's practice is to ask the mother and baby to attend one hour before the test session. The baby is given then a small dose of trimeprazine, fed and changed and usually, by the time of testing, is sleepy. The interesting results obtained in neonates are discussed later in this chapter.

The most easily identifiable response in the BER complex is the fifth wave (NV) that is so often inseparably merged with the fourth wave (NIV), and in particular, it is the positive-going limb of this response (FFP7) which can be clearly identified. The NV response occurs with a latency of about 6–7 ms in adults and 7.6 to 8.6 ms in babies. It can usually be identified after only a few hundred stimuli have been delivered.

The simplest method of checking that valid responses are being obtained is to concentrate initially on the NV alone. Begin by determining the 6 ms point on the analysis sweep of the averager and then deliver stimuli at 20–50 per second at 80 dB HL. The NV should be clearly visible after about 20 seconds in a hearing subject. The test then can be repeated and it should be possible to superimpose the two recordings. If the purpose of the test is to estimate auditory acuity, one gradually reduces the stimulus intensity, comparing each response with its predecessor, until NV can no longer be identified (Fig. 5.10). If a neuro-otological test is intended, one can alter the stimulus presentation rate to ten per second so that the earlier BER components may be more easily identified; the stimulus intensity may be maintained at a supra-threshold level, but more than one recording is required so that the consistency of the waves may be noted.

Recent clinical work

The clinical uses of BER may be divided conveniently into those estimating acuity and those attempting neuro-otological diagnosis.

As a measure of auditory acuity

Firstly, one must remember that this test measures the threshold of the auditory response at the level of the inferior colliculus and higher lesions may upset hearing without being detected by BER methods. Nevertheless, BER indicates the hearing threshold in the vast majority of cases.

The first wave or 6 ms response (NV or N4b) to a click or high frequency tone pip is an excellent audiometric indicator. Using a 4800 Hz tone pip, Davis and Hirsch (1975) report that the threshold of detectability is usually at or below 10 dB SL. Davis (1975) now routinely uses BER for the hearing evaluation of children but still employs the slow vertex ERA potential for the detection of threshold at lower frequencies. Schulman-Galambos and Galambos (1975), Suzuki (1975) and Mokotoff, Schulman Galambos and Galambos (1977) state that BER is recordable almost without exception from adults and infants as young as 33 weeks gestational age. Yamada (1975) shows how eight patients with

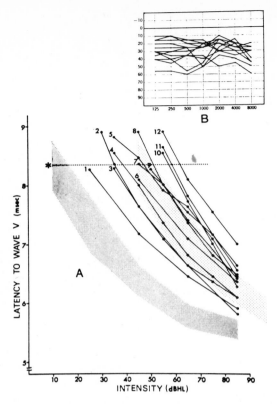

Fig. 5.11 The latency/intensity functions of the BER in 12 patients with conductive hearing losses. (Yamada *et al.* (1975), by permission *Auris. Nasus. Larynx.*).

a conductive hearing loss could be distinguished from normal subjects by the intensity/latency function of the fifth wave (Fig. 5.11). Patients with cochlear lesions often show an abnormally rapid change in both intensity/latency function and intensity/amplitude function which may be related to recruitment.

Sohmer and Tell (1975) reported a series of 20 patients with a suspected non-organic hearing loss who were successfully evaluated using BER. It may be that this method will prove ideal for evaluating claims of industrial hearing impairment.

As a means of neuro-otological diagnosis

The maturation of the auditory pathway in premature infants and neonates. BER provide an interesting electrophysiological correlate of auditory development. Jewett and Romano (1972) reported in rats and cats the gradual change in the profile of BER responses from birth over the following weeks until the adult waveform is reached in 1–2 months. Similar work was performed more recently by Buchwald and Huang (1975) in cats alone. Since BER are obtained by a non-invasive technique, they may be recorded from human neonates without fear of any legal or ethical problems. Hecox and Galambos (1974) have described the development of BER in human subjects and have shown how the waveform alters during the first few weeks of life (Fig. 5.12). At birth, the latency of the later waves is progressively more delayed compared to the adult BER and only the third and fifth waves are prominent. Over the next three months, the latency of each of the latter waves shortens until the waveform resembles that of an adult and gradually the other waves of the response become more prominent. More recently Salamy and McKean (1976) have conducted a similar study.

Schulman-Galambos and Galambos (1975) have investigated a series of 24 premature human infants and they found that BER were reliably obtained in every baby, even in one that was only of 34 weeks gestational age.

BER offer two clinical services for neonates: firstly, they offer a reliable screening test for auditory acuity which is harmless to apply; secondly, they may be used to assess the maturity of the infant. The future should bring reports of BER in various abnormalities such as hyperbilirubinaemia, mongolism, gargoylism, etc., and it is hoped it will extend our knowledge in these fields.

Multiple sclerosis.   Multiple sclerosis or disseminated sclerosis is a fairly common disorder affecting mainly young adults. The clinical picture is remarkable for its variation, the speed of progression varies from a few weeks to many years. Patchy plaques of demyelination occur in the white matter of the brain and spinal cord and lead to a variety of neurological signs: ocular disturbances, cerebellar ataxia, posterior column sensory loss, limb spasticity and mental changes are amongst the commoner features. Vertigo is very common whilst deafness is rare.

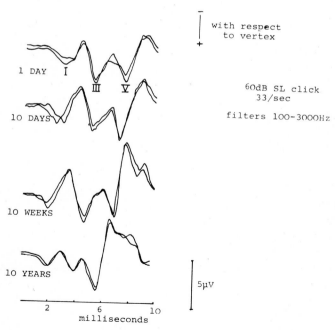

Fig. 5.12 Typical BER patterns recorded at different ages in normal subjects (Adapted from Schulman-Galambos, C. & Galambos, R. (1975)).

Robinson and Rudge (1975) interpreted thirty patients with multiple sclerosis. Several patients had internuclear ophthalmoplegia, but none revealed any hearing loss. Twenty-two of the group of 30 patients showed an abnormal delay of the later waves of the BER. It is interesting that they managed to obtain clear recordings after averaging only 512 responses using a click stimulus and filters 0.2 sec to 2.5 kHz. Halliday, McDonald and Mushin (1972) have shown a latency delay of the visual evoked response in cases of multiple sclerosis. Douek, Gibson and Humphries (1975) demonstrated similar changes using their 'crossed acoustic response' which records the post-aural myogenic responses from both sides of the head. Thornton and Hawkes (1976b) reported that virtually all the patients they tested with definite multiple sclerosis according to Schumacher's criteria gave responses which fell outside the normal amplitude/latency limits (see Fig. 5.6). All the patients had normal or near normal hearing. Robinson and Rudge (1977) believe that pairs of click stimuli 5ms apart, presented at a fast repetition rate stress the auditory system and make the abnormality of the V wave marked in multiple sclerosis.

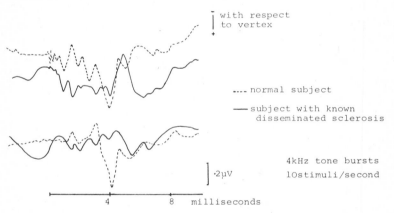

with respect to vertex

.... normal subject

—— subject with known disseminated sclerosis

·2µV

4kHz tone bursts
10 stimuli/second

4   8   milliseconds

Fig. 5.13 The ipsilateral and contralateral BER recorded from a young girl known to be suffering from disseminated sclerosis.

The author has found in a small series of 12 patients that often the NV response follows the N1 response by a latency gap of more than 5 ms. The contralateral-/ipsilateral recordings may show obvious differences when compared with normal subjects (Fig. 5.13).

It would appear that BER offers a sensitive test for the detection of demyelination within the brainstem.

Eighth nerve tumours. Four different BER findings have been reported that occur in patients with eighth nerve tumours.

1. *Loss of the BER waveform following NI.* Sohmer, Feinmesser and Szabo (1974) reported that on stimulating the affected ear of a patient with an eighth nerve tumour (acoustic neuroma), the BER waveform could only be traced as far as the site of the lesion and the N2, N3, N4 and N5 peaks were absent. Similar findings were reported by Starr and Hamilton (1976). Selters and Brackmann

(1977) have investigated a series of 100 patients clinically suspected of retrocochlear disorders and subsequent investigation showed that 36 had vestibulo-cochlear Schwannoma (acoustic neuroma), 10 had other retrocochlear tumours and 44 were tumour-free. These authors (Selters and Brackmann, 1977) reported that 46 per cent of the tumour group gave poorly-developed BER waveforms and the NV was unrecognisable. On five records, only NI was identifiable, and all these patients had 3–4 cm tumours located medially in the cerebro-pontine angle; four of the patients had excellent hearing on pure tone audiometry and one might have expected a smaller tumour size.

2. *Latency delay of NV.* Selters and Brackmann (1977) noted that 54 per cent of the tumour patients in their series had a recordable NV wave on stimulating the affected ear but this wave often showed a latency delay when compared with the NV produced on stimulating the normal ear. They (Selters and Brackmann, 1977) used an 83 dB HL click stimulus (160 μs electrical duration) and all the patients had pure tone hearing thresholds better than 75 dB average for 2, 4 and 8 kHz. A correction factor was often applied as the hearing thresholds between the normal and affected ears often differed. A latency delay of over 0.2 ms was believed to be significant if there was an auditory threshold difference of 0–50 dB, 0.3 ms with a difference of 50–65 dB and 0.4 ms with a difference of over 65 dB. Using these criteria, 96 per cent of tumour patients were successfully identified and 12 per cent of false positive diagnoses were reached.

3. *Differences between ipsilateral and contralateral recordings.* Thornton (1974) showed an abnormality of the first wave (N1) when recorded from the ipsilateral side of the head using binaural stimulation and suggested that careful examination of the traces might indicate that the stimulus entering only from the normal contralateral ear was travelling unhindered up the brainstem. He postulated that by comparing the recordings using bilateral and monaural stimulation, it may be possible further to localise the site of dysfunction.

4. *Latency delay between the NIII and NV peaks.* Selters and Brackmann (1977) measured the time elapsing between the NIII and NV peaks and found significant delays only in those patients with large (over 3 cm diameter) tumours. This may prove to be a useful means of predicting tumour size.

It may be concluded that BER shows promise in the early detection of eighth nerve tumours. Figure 5.14 shows the BER waveform from a patient with a large medially-placed eighth nerve tumour and a 90 dB hearing loss in the affected ear. The ECochG showed a normal AP configuration with a threshold of 70 dB HL.

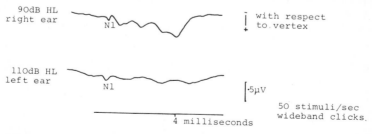

Fig. 5.14 The BER recorded from a subject with a large eighth nerve tumour affecting his left ear.

Only the NI of the BER on the affected side can be identified with certainty.

Midbrain tumours.   Starr and Achor (1975) and Starr and Hamilton (1976) have reported the BER findings in patients with various midbrain tumours. They found that the BER waveform could usually be identified to the level of the site of dysfunction, for instance, with tumours above the superior olivary complex the NI, NII and NIII were identified but the NIV and NV were absent.

Other central lesions.   Thornton (1974) reports a fascinating case of a diver in the Royal Navy who suffered 'the staggers', a vestibular form of decompression sickness during a deep dive using oxygen/helium mixture. The bubbles, released from the blood, are thought to cause microlesions within the brainstem. When first tested, the patient had a 35 dB 2 kHz audiometric loss and the BER showed an abnormally small N3 response and an absence of the sixth wave (NVI or N5). Six months later, his hearing improved to 15 dB at 2 kHz, the N3 was enlarged and the sixth wave was visible. One year later, his hearing now recovered to normal (5 dB at 2 kHz), his BER appeared to be within normal limits.

Comatosed patients.   Starr and Achor (1975) performed BER investigations on 37 comatosed patients with aetiologies that included drug overdoses, hypoxia, diabetic coma, hepatic failure and status epilepticus. The BER was not altered in respect of latency in any of the conditions. One woman patient gave a similar BER both when deep in coma and a few days later when she was conscious.

Brain death.   Starr and Achor (1975) have used BER to assess brain death in 20 cases. They found that typically only the first wave (N1) was obtainable.

Conclusions

Acoustic brainstem electrical responses (BER) are the most recent addition to the field of clinical ERA and, undoubtedly, they represent one of the most exciting advances.

The main advantages of BER are that they may be obtained using harmless, non-invasive electrodes and that sedatives do not affect the responses. The disadvantage of their small amplitude is easily overcome by averaging techniques as it is possible to use rapid stimulus presentation rates allowing the average of a very large number of responses to be taken.

BER provide an excellent means of estimating the hearing acuity in young children and babies, except in the low frequency domain. These responses seem destined to provide the paedo-audiologist with the necessary ERA back-up for his clinical skills.

The neuro-otological use of BER appears bright. Perhaps its use will appeal more to the neurologist than to the otologist because as no invasive technique is required, the test can be quite safely performed by non-otological workers.

6. The Myogenic (Sonomotor) Responses

All the muscles of the body react to sound (Bickford, Galbraith and Jacobson, 1963a; Bickford, Jacobson and Galbraith, 1963b). The muscles within the middle ear, particularly the stapedius muscle, contract in a consistent manner. The other muscles of the body, such as those of the arms and legs, only react in an inconsistent manner in response to intense sound stimulation although some of the muscles around the scalp may be excited by less intense sounds. The muscles behind the ear of an animal, such as a dog, can be actually seen to move but because these muscles are vestigial in man averaging techniques are required to enable the responses to be detected.

Although acoustically-evoked myogenic responses provide a fascinating field of study, the clinical application of the responses from muscles outside the tympanic cavity is doubted by many workers. There are, nevertheless, possible clinical uses for the post-auricular responses both as an approximate measure of hearing acuity and as a neuro-otological tool, so one particular method of recording these responses (the 'crossed acoustic method') is described later in this chapter.

Historically, myogenic responses were the first to be recorded using electronic averaging techniques. Geisler, Frishkopf and Rosenblith (1958) recorded responses to clicks from the scalp in human subjects. Initially they believed the responses to be neurogenic but it was clearly shown by Bickford *et al*. (1963a, 1963b) that the source was muscular and today little doubt exists. In 1964, Bickford, Jacobson and Cody, as well as Cody *et al*. (1964) showed how curare abolished all the fast responses (10–30 ms) with the exception of some components of the parietal response. Following these early days at least four different myogenic responses have attracted attention:

The *inion response* is obtained with the active electrode on or near the external occipital protuberance (inion) and is probably derived from the cervical musculature. Because it can be obtained from deaf patients with intact vestibular function (Cody *et al*., 1964; Gibson, 1974), it would be unwise to use the response to predict hearing acuity. Attempts to associate this response with the function of the vestibular semicircular canals has met with little success (Tabor *et al*., 1968; Pignatro, 1972), so Townsend and Cody (1971) have suggested a generator site in the saccule. The largest component of the response complex is negative at the inion with a peak latency of 30 ms.

The *post-auricular response* is obtained from an active electrode placed over the post-auricular muscles immediately behind the pinna. The response amplitude is reduced by 90 per cent if the electrode is placed more than 2 cm from the

133

optimum site (Vaughan and Ritter, 1970). The post-auricular response was first reported by Kiang *et al.* (1963) who noted its variability and habituation. The response complex varies according to the recording bandwidth limits (Thornton, 1975c) but it is generally reported that, with the active electrode on the post-auricular region, the largest components are negative with a peak latency of approximately 13 ms and with a following positive peak with a latency of 16 ms. Yoshie and Okudaira (1969) believed this response to be truly cochleo-myogenic and using click stimulation found that it could provide a measure of hearing acuity. In 1973, Douek, Gibson and Humphries reported their first clinical attempts to use the post-auricular responses as a means of 'objective audiometry' and noted the results from patients with various brainstem disorders.

The *parietal response* is a complex mixture of neurogenic and myogenic components. The main interest centres on the neurogenic elements which are believed to arise from the medial geniculate body and the primary auditory cortex. These responses are mentioned in detail in Chapter Eight.

The *acoustic jaw reflex* has been reported by Meir-Ewert, Gleitsmann and Reiter (1974). It can only be demonstrated if the chewing muscles are voluntarily activated and these workers believe that it represents an inhibition, or quiet period, of the on-going muscle activity. The reflex was absent in six patients with complete deafness and normal vestibular function, so the reflex arc probably involves the acoustic nerve alone. As it can only be elicited using intense sound stimulation, its application for estimating hearing acuity is doubtful.

At present, most work has been devoted to the post-aural myogenic response. This chapter will deal mainly with this response but will mention the other responses briefly.

Terminology

In the mid 1960's, all the acoustically-evoked responses which occurred with a latency of less than 50 ms were described as 'the fast responses'. Since then a number of quite different 'fast responses' have been introduced into ERA (ECochG, BER, early cortical responses, etc.) and so a further classification is necessary. Davis (1965a) has suggested the excellent term 'sonomotor responses' which may be used to describe all the various myogenic responses including the inion response which is not necessarily cochleo-motor. The different sonomotor responses can then be described according to the active electrode site: e.g., post-auricular sonomotor response. This terminology is now well established and fortunately not controversial.

Douek, Gibson and Humphries (1973) wished to stress their particular method of obtaining the post-auricular sonomotor response. They used electrodes placed at specific positions close to the muscle mass on each side and then recorded the responses simultaneously from both sides. To avoid the term 'bilateral simultaneously-evoked post-auricular sonomotor responses' which they thought unwieldy, they introduced the term 'crossed acoustic response'. The term is easily criticised, however, as it may lead the reader to believe that the response is only obtained from behind the contralateral ear whereas it is a bilateral response.

Further confusion has been added as Jerger, Neely and Jerger (1975) have used the same term to describe the intra-tympanic acoustic reflex when obtained from the opposite ear to the stimulus.

Anatomy and physiology

The sonomotor responses are reflexes. A reflex act is often defined as the response resulting from the passage of nervous impulses through a reflex arc. A reflex arc consists of a chain of neurones linking the receptor which receives the stimulus (the afferent pathway) to the effector which acts to form the response (the efferent pathway). In the case of sonomotor responses, sound stimulates the receptor placed in the inner ear and the nervous impulses pass through the brainstem to reach a muscle group which effects the response.

One of the characteristics of muscle reflexes, e.g. the quadriceps stretch reflex or knee jerk, is that they fatigue. The latent period between the stimulus and the response becomes prolonged and the rise of tension smaller and more gradual. Reflex fatigue is due to some change developing in the central pathway; thus, when a stretch reflex can no longer be elicited, direct stimulation of the peripheral nerve still results in muscular contraction. The intimate nature of central fatigue of reflexes is unknown but it is known that when the blood supply of the reflex centre is impaired, or if it is depressed with anaesthetics, fatigue occurs sooner. This characteristic of muscle reflexes has been found to be typical of the sonomotor responses and to be the cause of most of the recording difficulties.

The anatomical pathway of each of the sonomotor responses may be divided for descriptive purposes into an afferent pathway which is usually the cochlea and auditory nerve, a central pathway which passes through synapses in various nuclei of the brainstem and an efferent pathway which involves the appropriate peripheral nerve and muscles which effect the response. An indication of the central pathway can be obtained by considering the onset latency of each response. The time taken for the response to reach the cochlear nucleus can be assumed by considering the onset latency of the second BER response, and the time taken for the response to pass along the peripheral nerve to the neuromuscular junction and for the muscle to react can also be fairly easily calculated. If one then subtracts the time spent in both the peripheral pathways from the total onset latency of the response, the latency of the central pathway is obtained. The delay passing along the central pathway is mainly accounted for by the number of synapses—obviously the time taken to cross a synapse varies with intensity but in general it is approximately 0.7 ms at 80 dB SPL (Totsuka, Nakamura and Kirkae, 1954).

The post-auricular response. Most evidence suggests that this response is generated by the cochlea and then travels to the cochlear nucleus; the latency for this pathway is approximately 2.4 ms. The response finally leaves the brainstem along the facial nerve to reach the post-aural muscles; the length of nerve involved is about 5–7 cm the conduction velocity is about 50 metres/sec, and the impulse takes about 0.7 ms to cross the neuromuscular junction. Thus one may calculate that the time taken for the post-aural response to travel along its peripheral pathways is approximately 5.2 ms. As the onset latency of the response is about 8 ms, the latency of the central pathway is approximately 2.8 ms and must therefore involve 4 synapses.

Direct evidence about the central pathway in man is lacking because human experimentation is clearly not feasible. Some animals, such as the cat and guinea pig, have well developed sonomotor post-auricular responses which are often called the Preyer reflex (Preyer, 1881). Totsuka et al. (1954) have traced the pathway of Preyer's reflex in the cat. As the latency of the response in the cat is only 4.8 ms, it is uncertain how these cat results compare with man in whom the latency is 8 ms, but the difference may partly be explained by the greater length of the peripheral pathway. In the cat, the response involves the superior olivary complex and the lateral lemniscus, and it would not be surprising if a similar pathway existed in man. It is not known whether the human pathway reaches as high as the inferior colliculus, but it is unlikely to involve the cerebellum as Sohmer (1973) has recorded a post-auricular response from an anencephalic premature infant in whom autopsy revealed no cerebellar development. Galambos (1956a) favoured the theory that sonomotor acoustic responses involve synapses actually within the reticular formation. The reticular formation is an anatomically ill-defined area of the brainstem lying close to the mid-line which has functions that are intimately related to the state of muscle tone and general alertness. The post-auricular response is certainly very sensitive to such factors, so it is quite possible that synapses do lie in this area. It is also known that, at each synapse within the CNS, there are other nerve endings not directly concerned with the passage of the response which have inhibitory or excitatory functions. Even if there is no actual synapse in the reticular formation, it is more than likely that this structure influences the passage of the response through the brainstem.

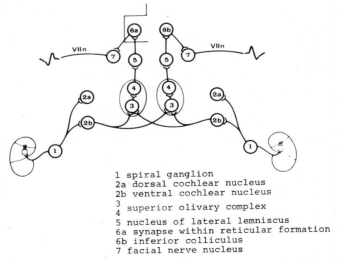

1 spiral ganglion
2a dorsal cochlear nucleus
2b ventral cochlear nucleus
3
4 superior olivary complex
5 nucleus of lateral lemniscus
6a synapse within reticular formation
6b inferior colliculus
7 facial nerve nucleus

Fig. 6.1 The probable neural pathway of the post-aural sonomotor response (Gibson (1974), by permission London University).

Considering the anatomical pathways available and the latency of the post-auricular response together with the known experimental findings in the cat, the most likely central pathway in man is: ventral cochlear nucleus—superior olivary complex—a second synapse with the superior olivary complex—the nucleus of the lateral lemniscus—reticular formation or inferior colliculus—facial nerve nucleus (Fig. 6.1).

At present, this suggested pathway is highly speculative but it is hoped that as more patients with known brainstem lesions are tested, some of the mysteries will be solved.

The other sonomotor responses.   It is likely that a fairly similar central pathway exists for all the sonomotor responses but that the latency varies because of differences in the different peripheral pathways. The generator site for the inion response is not yet known with certainty but it seems to involve both cochlear and vestibular receptors.

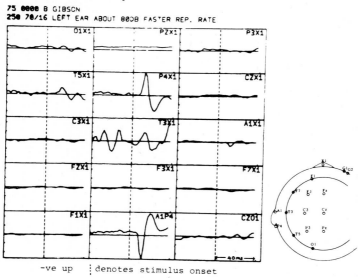

Fig. 6.2 The electrical activity recorded simultaneously from various scalp positions during click stimulation (Gibson (1974), by permission *London University*).

Some characteristics of the responses

The electrode positions

Myogenic responses can be recorded from many parts of the scalp. Figure 6.2 shows the responses obtained from various electrode positions. The inion response is just visible on the CZ 01 recording and has peak latency of 30 ms (this particular subject has a clear post-aural response which is even obtained from the earlobe to nasion recording).

The best active electrode site for the post-aural response lies close to the attachment of the pinna to the scalp over the main bulk of the post-aural muscle (Kiang *et al.*, 1963; Yoshie and Okudaira, 1967). If one wishes to localise the

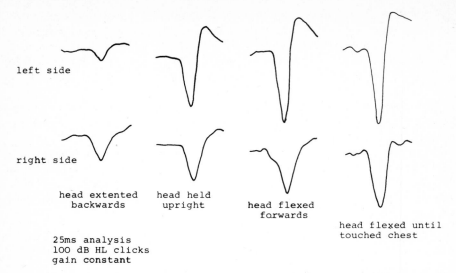

Fig. 6.3 Alterations of the post-auricular response caused by flexing and extending the neck. The subject was a young adult who gave clear, consistent responses.

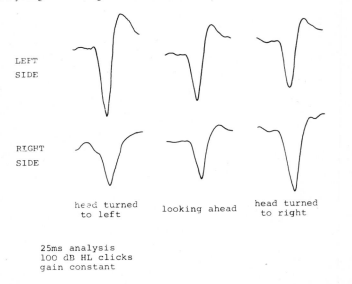

Fig. 6.4 Alterations of the post-auricular response caused by turning the head. The subject was a young adult who gave clear, consistent responses.

response to this muscle alone, it helps to place the 'reference' electrode close to the muscle without any other intervening muscle groups. Gibson (1974) found that a 'reference' electrode on the earlobe gave a marginally larger response than one placed on the neck but that the neck placement was easier in active young children.

The inion sonomotor response is best obtained by placing the active electrode on the scalp immediately over the inion. A 'reference' electrode can be placed on the earlobe.

The bilateral nature of the post-aural response

If one ear is stimulated alone, post-aural sonomotor responses can be recorded from behind both ears. This property was first noted by Kiang *et al.* (1963). The contralateral response is not due to cross talk or lack of masking; bilateral responses can be obtained in patients with total unilateral hearing losses on stimulating the hearing ear; the contralateral response can be obtained when the opposite ear is adequately masked and the latency of the contralateral response is within ± 2 ms of that of the ipsilateral response in normal subjects (Gibson, 1974).

The effect of changes in muscle tone

All sonomotor responses are extremely sensitive to changes in muscle tone. Bickford *et al.* (1963a, 1963b) noted that the inion response was enhanced by increasing flexion of the neck and that it was often totally abolished by extending the neck. Kiang *et al.* (1963) found soon after discovering the post-aural response that its amplitude varied on adopting various head positions. The effect of flexion and extension of the neck on the post-aural response is shown in Figure 6.3. The effect of turning the head from left to right is shown in Figure 6.4 and it is interesting to note that the response from behind the left ear is enhanced and the response from behind the right ear is diminished by turning the head to the left, and vice versa; this illustrates the importance of obtaining the response bilaterally if it is to be used for hearing prediction in young children.

Muscle relaxants affect all the sonomotor responses. Cody *et al.* (1964) were unable to obtain the responses from a curarised patient who was fully conscious. Graham, Hutton and Beagley (1975) have also shown the loss of the post-auricular response after administering a muscle relaxant during general anaesthesia. Gibson (1974) found that tranquillising drugs and alcohol diminished the post-aural response.

If a subject can voluntarily contract his post-aural muscles, large post-aural sonomotor responses are obtained. Jacobson *et al.* (1964) found that, if the branch of the facial nerve supplying the post-aural muscles was blocked by the injection of a local anaesthetic, no post-aural responses could be recorded.

The effect of subject attention

Although it is found that larger sonomotor responses are obtained when the subject is in an attentive state, this is merely because of enhanced muscle tone and definitely not because of any direct cortical influence. If the subject grows bored and his muscle tone diminishes, the responses become very difficult to identify.

The optimum stimulus characteristics

Studies show that the post-aural response is evoked by change in stimulus state and that if a pure tone burst is employed, a post-aural response may be obtained both at the onset and the conclusion of the burst. Generally, it appears that it is the onset of the stimulus which evokes the sonomotor response and that the rise time is critical (Gibson, 1974). Figure 6.5 shows the effect of varying the rise time

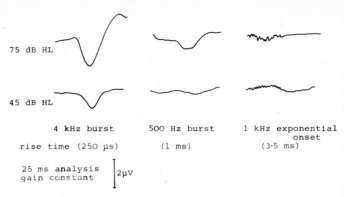

Fig. 6.5 Alterations of the post-auricular response caused by varying the rise-time of the stimulus.

of the stimulus in four normal subjects. A fast rise time, preferably less than $250\,\mu s$, is essential if the post-aural responses are to be obtained using low intensities, and this may explain why Cody and Bickford (1969) were unable to record responses at low intensities in the majority of their subjects using a pure tone burst of 1 kHz, whilst Yoshie and Okudaira (1969) found the responses to clicks indicated the psychophysical threshold in nearly all of their subjects. Unfortunately, the necessity for a fast stimulus rise time limits the use of post-aural responses in the low frequency domain (less than 1 kHz) (Douek, Gibson and Humphries, 1975).

The recovery functions of the post-aural response

The post-aural response recovers rapidly and Kiang *et al.* (1963) identified responses using click stimulus repetition rates in excess of 200 per second. Yoshie and Okudaira (1969) in a detailed investigation showed that full recovery of the response occurs after an interstimulus interval of 140 ms and that the response

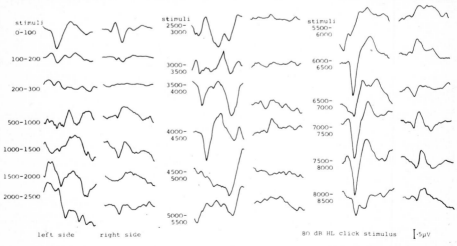

Fig. 6.6 The effect of continuous stimulation (10 per second) on the post-auricular response from one subject.

has recovered 90 per cent of its amplitude within 100 ms. It would appear that a stimulus repetition rate of 10 per second is reasonable for most purposes.

The effect of prolonged or repeated stimulation (habituation)

The literature varies widely on the subject of the effects of prolonged stimulation on the sonomotor responses. Davis et al. (1963) reported that the post-aural response habituates rapidly. Jacobson et al. (1964) stated that there is no evidence of fatigue or habituation. Kiang et al. (1963) found the post-aural response exasperating as patients appeared to become conditioned and then fail to yield responses. This latter group of workers reported that the response can be 'revived' by giving the subject an electric shock to his feet. Figure 6.6 shows the responses obtained from one subject to a click stimulus presented at a rate of 10 per second during a 15 minute period. The response is unidentifiable after only 200 stimuli but reappears after 1500 stimuli. The response then disappears again to reappear after 4000 stimuli. After 6000 stimuli the largest responses are seen and they last until 8000 stimuli have been presented before the response diminishes once more. These findings are typical of a study undertaken by the author and may account for some of the confusion in the literature. The most likely explanation is that the size of the response is chiefly dependent on the amount of muscle tone and that this varies with the subject's alertness during the test period. Certainly, the responses always immediately increases in size when the subject was asked to perform a task regardless of the extent of preceding stimulation.

The responses obtained on repeatedly testing the subject after short rest

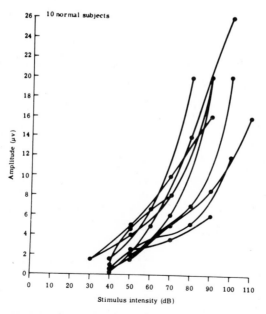

Fig. 6.7 The amplitude/intensity graph of the post-auricular response in normal subjects (Gibson (1974), by permission *London University*).

periods are identical to those obtained using continuous periods of stimulation. It appears to be essential that the subject's interest should be maintained throughout a test session and that he must not be allowed to relax. The relaxation of muscle tone is easily identifiable as the peak to peak amplitude of the on-going recording decreases—at this point the test must be abandoned until the subject has been 'enlivened'. Fortunately, young children rarely relax during a short test period and problems in maintaining muscle tone rarely arise.

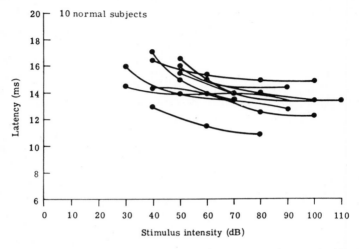

Fig. 6.8 The latency/intensity functions of the post-auricular response in normal subjects (Gibson, (1974), by permission *London University*).

Effects of altering the stimulus intensity

Amplitude and intensity functions. The amplitude of the response is most easily measured as the difference in μV between the peak of the main negative deflection at approximately 12 ms and the peak of the ensuing positive deflection. Yoshie and Okudaira (1969) remarked that the growth of the amplitude with increasing stimulus intensity was exponential, but caution in interpreting the results is needed as the response was very variable. Gibson (1974) plotted the amplitude/intensity functions for 10 normally-hearing adult subjects who gave clear responses and found similar results to those already reported (Fig. 6.7).

Latency and intensity functions. Gibson (1974) also recorded the latency of the main negative peak with regard to the stimulus onset as timed at the tympanic membrane (Fig. 6.8). It may be noted that as the stimulus intensity decreases, the latency of the response becomes prolonged. The latency/intensity functions of the post-aural sonomotor response is similar in rate of change to the latency/intensity functions of the cells of the superior olivary complex.

Effect of altering bandwidth recording limits

The power spectrum of a post-aural response has been analysed by Thornton (1975c) who reported that the main spectral peak is at about 600 Hz and that the spectrum extends from approximately 100 Hz to 1600 Hz. When a wide band recording system is used the post-auricular response comprises a complex of five peaks (P1 10ms, N1 12ms, P2 15ms, N2 19.5ms, P3 24ms). If the low pass filter is set at 200 Hz, the recording becomes much quieter as much of the background activity is rejected and the N1 and P3 components predominate. There is some advantage in limiting the low pass filter in this manner in active young children, as it makes identification of responses simpler.

The sensory receptor of the sonomotor responses

It is essential to know whether a sonomotor response is generated by stimulation of cochlear, vestibular or tactile receptors.

The post-aural response.   Kiang *et al.* (1963) reported that they were unable to obtain post-aural myogenic responses in any of the deaf patients that they tested. Most other workers believe that the post-aural response can only be obtained by cochlear stimulation (Bochenek and Bochenek (1975)). Gibson (1974) tested 11 patients who had total deafness in one or both ears and was unable to obtain a post-aural response. He found also that the response was not affected by absence of a caloric response (Hallpike-FitzGerald bithermal testing) and he could find no evidence of any tactile origin. Odenthal and Eggermont (1974), however, have recorded a possible post-aural myogenic response from one subject during electrocochleography, but this appears to be the only case mentioned in the literature.

The inion response.   This response shows many peculiarities. It can definitely be recorded from some totally deaf subjects in whom caloric tests reveal functioning cristae in the lateral semicircular canal but attempts to assess vestibular function using the inion response have failed, as it cannot always be evoked in such subjects. A possible explanation is that the inion response may originate from another part of the vestibular apparatus, and both Gibson (1974) and Townsend and Cody (1971) have suggested the saccule. Bickford (1966) has also obtained the inion response to tactile stimulation. It would appear that the inion sonomotor response may be evoked by stimulation of either cochlear, vestibular or tactile receptors.

The variability of the responses

The amplitude, latency and shape of the sonomotor responses vary considerably. Not only are there variations between different subjects but also between responses obtained from the same subject on different days or even after shorter intervals. Most of these changes can be related to muscle tone but, perhaps they can also be related to the individual variation in the bulk of the muscle available to generate the response. The post-aural muscles are vestigial and the amount of muscle present varies from subject to subject—some subjects invariably give only small responses and rarely can they voluntarily move their ears.

An illustration of the extreme variability of the post-aural response is shown in Figure 6.9. It may be seen that many of the responses are of minute amplitude, 36 per cent being under $2 \mu V$ at 80 dB SL. Gibson (1974) found it impossible to trace such small responses down to within 30 dB of the psycho-acoustic threshold. The situation is improved if the responses obtained from both sides of the head simultaneously are considered; if only the side of the head yielding the larger

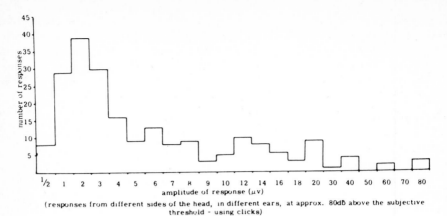

(responses from different sides of the head, in different ears, at approx. 80dB above the subjective threshold - using clicks)

Fig. 6.9 Variations in the amplitude of the post-auricular response encountered on testing a large number of subjects. Some subjects had normal hearing and most had some hearing loss. (Gibson (1974), by permission *London University*).

response amplitude is considered, then only 22 per cent of the responses are under $2 \mu V$ and none are under $1 \mu V$. It is not, however, predictable which side of the head will yield the greater response.

The shape of the post-aural sonomotor responses varies between subjects but the most consistent peak is the N1 occurring at about 13 ms. The latency of the response is the most stable feature and varies by only ± 3 ms in 98 per cent of a large group of normal subjects (Gibson, 1974). The latency of a large amplitude response is always shorter by 1 or 2 ms than when the muscles have 'fatigued' and yield a smaller amplitude of response to the same stimulus.

The detection of sonomotor responses at low stimulus intensities

Yoshie and Okudaira (1969) have suggested that the post-aural sonomotor response may be used as a means of estimating the psycho-acoustic hearing threshold. Gibson (1974) found that if a click stimulus was used (rise time 250 μ sec), a post-aural response could be detected from that side of the head yielding the larger response in 92 per cent of subjects using intensities within 30 dB of their hearing threshold for the same stimulus. Thornton (1975d) reported that the mean post-auricular sonomotor threshold vs. audiometric threshold was 9 dB with only 7 dB standard deviation. These figures appear to be quite different from those obtained by Cody and Bickford (1969) but these workers were using a less favourable stimulus.

The inion response may also be obtained using intensities close to the audiometric threshold, but because of its possible generation by tactile and vestibular receptors, it has not recently been used by any workers as a means of estimating auditory acuity.

The frequency specificity of the responses

The requirement of a fast stimulus rise time, needed to evoke consistent responses, makes it difficult to use stimuli of 1 kHz or lower frequency presented as pure tone bursts. Frequency specificity cannot be obtained using filtered clicks as it is found that the sharp transient at the onset of such a stimulus evokes the response (Douek *et al.*, 1975). Admittedly, some subjects are encountered with large sonomotor responses in whom low frequency tone bursts do evoke satisfactory response, but these subjects are few.

The test and test/retest reliability

The reliability of the post-aural sonomotor responses has already been mentioned and it is only necessary to summarise the details. The post-auricular response does not provide a precise means of estimating the auditory threshold as the response is too variable. Using the 'crossed acoustic method' and click stimulation, it is possible to identify the response from at least one side of the head at 30 dB SL in 92 per cent of subjects. Occasionally, the response can not be obtained using stimuli of less than 60 dB SL intensity. The possibility of encountering a child who gives poor responses which do not relate closely to his hearing levels, means the post-auricular response can only be used as a crude indicator of hearing status.

The test/retest reliability of the post-auricular response is poor. It varies considerably in amplitude from one moment to the next during the same test session. Most of the amplitude changes can be related to loss of muscle tone. The latency does not vary much although it may become slightly prolonged, by one to two milliseconds, when a response diminishes greatly in amplitude. The largest responses are usually encountered at the start of a test period when the subject is fully alert. The post-auricular response also varies considerably, especially in amplitude, between one test session and the next. In general, subjects who give large responses tend to always give large responses; whilst subjects who give small responses on the first test seem always to give small responses on later testing.

Instrumentation

The instrumentation and testing procedure which will be described relate to recording the post-aural sonomotor response and in particular to the method described by Humphries, Gibson and Douek (1976) for recording the 'crossed acoustic response'. The 'crossed acoustic method' implies a technique of obtaining both the contralateral and ipsilateral post-aural response simultaneously so that the side giving the larger response can be selected or so that the responses from each side can be compared.

The basic apparatus required is similar to that described in Chapter 2 and only the special requirements for recording the 'crossed acoustic response' are listed.

The test environment

Subjects do not give clear responses if they relax, so they are best tested seated on a hard wooden chair. The test chamber must be large enough to accommodate not only a child but the mother and a worker who can supervise the test. The room does not need to be sound proof but should be quiet, as this test is not wholly accurate but only gives an indication of the hearing acuity to within 30 dB. Adults are usually tested wearing earphones. Children often will not tolerate earphones and are therefore tested using a free-field loudspeaker which should be placed as close as is convenient to the child's head. (It should not be forgotten that the intensity of sound varies inversely with distance and careful calibration is necessary.)

The stimulus generation

The stimulus requirements.   It has already been emphasised that the optimum stimulus is brief with a very rapid rise time. Clicks evoke excellent responses and pure tone bursts of 8–2 kHz of one sinewave rise time and two sine waves duration can be used to obtain some frequency specificity in the higher frequency range.

The stimulus repetition rate.   The most useful rate for clinical work is ten per second. The response should be visible within 15 seconds. Prolonged periods of stimulation, of two minutes or more, will always include the effect of a fatigue of the response in the averaged recording.

Stimulus transducer.   A high quality transducer is essential. No matter how rapid the onset of a click electrically, its acoustic waveform has a rise time which is chiefly dependent on the limitations of the transducer. An electrostatic speaker is a considerable advantage, especially if children are to be tested. Good quality earphones are used whenever monaural information is sought, but it is always necessary to mask the opposite ear at high stimulus intensities. The stimulus intensity may be calibrated in 10 dB steps.

Masking facilities.   Provisions for masking is essential. Narrow band masking can be used if pure tone bursts are employed. Clicks contain a wide spectrum of frequencies and are best masked using wide band noise.

The recording equipment

Electrodes.   Sonomotor responses may be recorded using either surface electrodes or needle electrodes placed through the skin directly into the muscles. Any good quality EEG electrodes may be used; most workers employ the standard EEG silver/silver chloride dome-shaped disc electrodes.

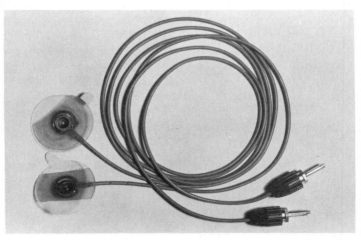

Fig. 6.10 The electrodes used for the 'crossed acoustic test'.

The crossed acoustic method of obtaining the post-auricular responses allows the use of electrodes placed within plastic shells which can be simply attached to the skin, often without the need for abraiding the underlying surface (Fig. 6.10). There is no need to glue the electrodes into position as they are placed outside the hairbearing region, and can be pressed simply into place using adhesive discs.

Amplifiers.   If the crossed acoustic method is to be used, it is essential that low noise biological amplifiers are used with a very high input impedance ($>$ 1000 MΩ) and a high common mode rejection ratio ($>$ 120 dB). Usually the pre-amplifier with a fixed gain is placed close to the subject and the final gain adjustment is made using the main amplifier which is housed with the averager. The total gain required varies between 10^4–10^5. Clarke (1976) has devised a small pre-amplifier which can be attached with a harness to the back of the child allowing him greater mobility. It has also been suggested that the input from each side of the head can be mixed together and fed as one signal to the main amplifier when the post-auricular response is used to obtain threshold information from children. (Douek and Clarke, 1976).

Filter settings (bandwidth).   The choice of narrow bandwidth settings facilitates the ease of identification of the main components of the post-auricular response, by eliminating a good deal of the background noise. Humphries *et al*. (1976) used a bandwidth of 1–200 Hz. Thornton (1975c) has shown that the use of a narrow bandwidth leads to considerable distortion of the post-auricular sonomotor response and to loss of identification of several of its components.

The averager.   Small purpose-built averagers are adequate for recording the post-auricular response. A single channel averager is sufficient for the 'crossed acoustic method' when threshold information alone is sought, as the input from each side of the head may be mixed. The use of a two channel averager is essential if neuro-otological work is to be performed and can be an advantage in testing children, as each channel provides a control against an artefact being mistaken for a true response; the response from one side of the head should occur within $\pm$ 2 ms of the other. Unfortunately, a two channel averager is expensive and may be beyond the financial reach of many smaller clinics.

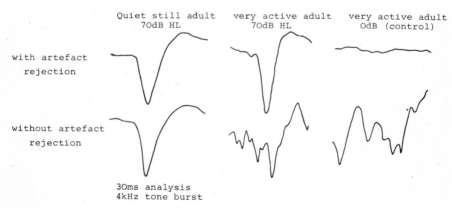

Fig. 6.11 Recordings of the post-auricular response showing the advantage of using an artefact rejection system.

The monitor oscilloscope.   It is most helpful to have a means of assessing the on-going background myogenic activity during recording sessions. If a subject relaxes, this background activity is low and the likelihood of obtaining a reasonable response considerably reduced. In these circumstances some mano-euvre must be employed to 'enliven' the subject or the test may have to be abandoned.

Artefact rejection facilities.   When the 'crossed acoustic method' is used to assess children, it is essential to have some means of rejecting sudden high voltage transient potentials which are generated by movements, or the averager will be overloaded with random activity making identification of the responses too hazardous for any practical value. Figure 6.11 shows the effect of using a simple system which rejects any transient signals exceeding a preset voltage level. Full details of a suitable system are given by Humphries *et al.* (1976).

Permanent recording of results.   These are clearly essential as with any method of ERA and details of possible systems are given in Chapter 2.

Testing procedures

The application of the 'crossed acoustic method' for obtaining the post-auricular sonomotor responses varies according to whether the test is applied to young children to estimate their hearing acuity or to adults for neuro-otological purposes.

Young children.   The main indication for using the 'crossed acoustic method' is the assessment of the hearing status of young children who are difficult to test using other methods. This technique can be applied within a few minutes to gain an approximate indication of the hearing acuity using clicks or high frequency tone bursts. Most normally-hearing children (approximately 80 per cent) yield

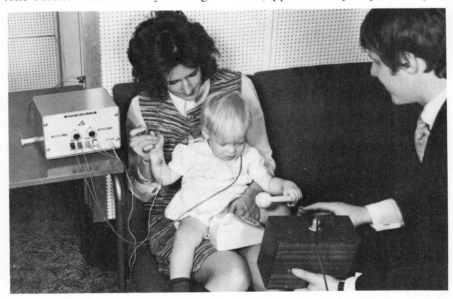

Fig. 6.12 A small child being tested using the 'crossed acoustic test' (Gibson (1974), by permission *London University*).

clear responses of over $2\,\mu$V amplitude to a stimulus of 80 dB HL so it is possible to identify smaller responses within 40 dB of their hearing threshold. Children with recruiting forms of hearing impairment also usually yield clear responses which 'collapse' rapidly as their threshold is approached. If no response can be identified, the child either has a hearing impairment or is a 'poor responder', and the finding has to be compared with the findings on behavioural or subjective testing. This test does not give an absolute indication of hearing impairment and is only useful when used together with other methods.

The children must not be sedated, as this may abolish the response. The main advantage of the method is that it can be applied to active young children even when there is some resistance to the test. If a child is too passive, the possibility of poor responses is increased and some other ERA technique may be better employed.

At Guy's Hospital, London where this test is used routinely, the child is first assessed by standard behavioural methods and then immediately sent for the 'crossed acoustic test'. The child may be apprehensive, so younger children are tested seated on their mothers' laps (Fig. 6.12). This not only gives the child some security but also allows the adult to control the movements of the child's arms. The electrodes are simply pressed into position after the skin has been cleaned with acetone. The active electrode is placed on the mastoid surface immediately behind the attachment of the pinna and the reference electrode is placed on the surface of the neck immediately below the tip of the same mastoid. Electrodes are placed on both sides of the head and each pair is directed into a different channel of the averager. The earth electrode is usually placed on the child's arm. Sometimes there is a brief struggle during the attachment of the electrodes, but once they are in position they are well-tolerated. It is possible to scratch the surface of the skin through the electrode when the electrode/skin impedance is high without upsetting the child. If the electrodes are accidentally removed during the test, the wide contact area usually provides sufficient adhesion to allow them to be pressed back into position.

The test period is generally limited to ten minutes, to avoid fatigue. Stimuli at 80 dB HL and 50 dB HL are delivered as a minimum using both clicks and a high frequency tone burst to gather the basic information, and then further intensities may be used according to the specific case.

Immediately after the test, the child is seen again in the assessment clinic where the results of behavioural and objective testing can be compared. In one series of 200 cases, disagreement in the results obtained by these two methods only occurred in six cases (Gibson, 1974).

Adults and older children.   Co-operative subjects are simply tested sitting on a fairly uncomfortable chair without any head support. The real problem in such cases is in maintaining active muscle tone, for when the subject relaxes the responses diminish dramatically. The tester has to ask the subject questions after each response has been obtained and to keep giving instructions to move the head forwards or grit the teeth, etc.

Neonates.   Ashcroft, Humphries and Douek (1975) have used the 'crossed acoustic method' to assess neonates and premature infants. These subjects do appear to possess adequate muscle tone to provide clear responses in the majority of cases. Because the method is simple and atraumatic, it raises no ethical problems and may provide a useful method of screening.

Identification of the post-aural response

The response is most easily identified by the negative peak which occurs with a latency of approximately 12–15 ms with respect to the arrival of the stimulus at the ear under test. Adults usually yield a response with a similar latency from both sides of the head which makes identification simple. Children may twist their heads so that the response may only be identified on one side and care has to be taken not to confuse any random muscle activity which has penetrated the barrier provided by the artefact rejection system. Often several trials must be collected before the response can be identified with certainty and in these circumstances the latency of each response is identical although the amplitude varies. It is certainly helpful to examine the response during averaging so that sudden changes can be noted and discounted. Hazell *et al.* (1977) have recently reported excellent results in using the postauricular response as a screening test for children by using a machine scoring method. It may well prove that machine scoring has significant advantages in this type of audiometry.

The clinical use of myogenic responses

A. The post-aural responses

The true clinical value of the post-aural responses is debatable but certain observations have been made using clinical material.

As a measure of auditory acuity

For the adult or co-operative subject, this response provides the least reliable

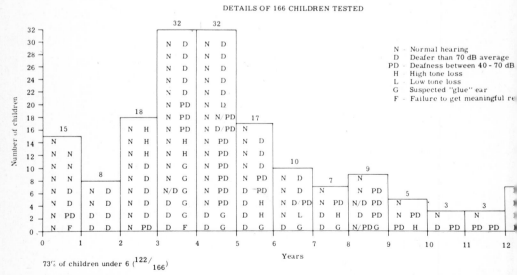

Fig. 6.13 Details of children tested using the 'crossed acoustic test' (Gibson (1974), by permission of *London University*).

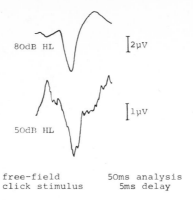

80dB HL

$\int$2µV

50dB HL

$\int$1µV

free-field   50ms analysis
click stimulus   5ms delay

Fig. 6.14 The post-auricular response from a mentally-retarded child who was very difficult to test by conventional means.

indication of the auditory threshold of all the ERA methods mentioned in this book. Its use is confined to providing an approximate measure in young alert children or neonates. The stimulus must either be a click or a tone burst at a frequency of 2 kHz or more, so it does not provide any indication of low frequency hearing. Figure 6.13 shows the results obtained using the 'crossed acoustic method' in 166 children without any sedation. Several of these children had been deemed unmanageable and behavioural assessment was almost impossible. The responses from one such case are shown in Figure 6.14. Only two children were impossible to test using this method and ten of the children gave only very limited information. The accuracy of these results has been assessed by various methods including transtympanic electrocochleography and only two serious errors have been known to have occurred. In conclusion, the test is of some value in ascertaining the hearing status of children. It should only be used in conjunction with other forms of testing because, being a muscle response, it is not always consistent. As an initial screening test it takes little time and places no great demands on the child.

As a means of neuro-otological diagnosis

The potential use of the post-aural response as a neuro-otological tool is somewhat marred by the lack of reliability and reproducibility which is so characteristic of sonomotor responses. Nevertheless, studies are possible in the majority of patients who do yield clear responses.

Conductive hearing losses. It has been noted (Gibson, 1974) that the post-aural responses obtained on stimulating an ear with a conductive hearing loss are smaller than those obtained from the normal ear using the same level of stimulus intensity. An example of a patient with a tympanic perforation is shown in Figure 6.15. It may be seen that the input-output functions of the affected ear resemble those from the normal ear except that they lie at higher stimulus intensities. In fact, if the graph was calibrated in terms of the sensation level (dB SL), the two ears would appear to be almost identical in their input-output functions. A similar observation is noted in other methods of ERA.

Children with sero-mucinous otitis media ('glue ears') tend to yield poor

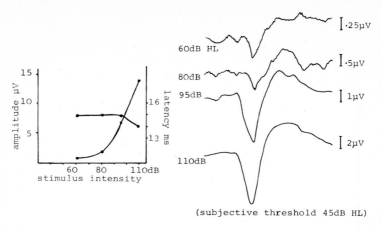

Fig. 6.15 The post-auricular responses and input/output functions from a subject with a conductive hearing loss (otosclerosis).

response (Gibson, 1974). This is due to the slow growth of the amplitude-intensity functions as noted in the previous paragraph. It is also found that the form of the response in many cases is broader than normal. Perhaps this latter finding is due to attenuation of the rapid onset of the click stimulus by the 'glue' into a stimulus with less favourable onset characteristics.

Probable cochlear hearing losses.   The post-auricular response has been examined in several patients who suffered from the phenomenon of recruitment. The presence of recruitment is almost diagnostic of a cochlear defect, as it is only rarely noted in cases with retro-cochlear pathological conditions (Dix, Hallpike and Hood, 1948).

It is found that patients with monaural recruiting hearing losses often give a response with as large an amplitude from the affected ear as from the normal ear when stimuli are delivered at high intensities (Fig. 6.16). This implies that it is dangerous to guess the hearing acuity of a subject after merely obtaining one response from an ear and it is always necessary to trace the responses 'down-

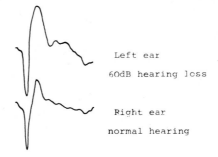

Fig. 6.16 The post-auricular responses from a subject with a 'recruiting' hearing loss. Note that the response from the abnormal ear is larger than that from the normally-earing ear.

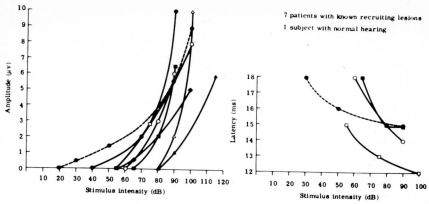

Fig. 6.17 The amplitude/intensity functions (left) and the latency/intensity functions (right) from patients with 'recruiting' hearing losses (Gibson (1974), by permission *London University*).

wards' using less and less intense stimulation until a response threshold is reached.

Most patients with recruiting hearing losses give clear responses and it is simple to construct input-output graphs (Fig. 6.17). The growth of the response amplitude with increasing stimulus intensity appears to be abnormally rapid in the presence of recruitment and may be compared to the psychophysical sensation of loudness in these cases. The latency functions show interesting changes but in several of the patients it is not possible to be sure of the exact position of the peak of the response. In some patients, especially those with Ménière's disorder, the latencies do not progressively lengthen as the stimulus intensity is reduced and jumps in latency or even shorter latencies occur. In those patients who do give clear and consistent changes in latency, the common finding is that the latency functions alter more rapidly than in patients with normal hearing or conductive lesions. This is the opposite of the effect that recruitment has on the latency functions in electrocochleography in which the latency change is less than in a normal ear. It would appear, therefore, that the latency change of the post-aural responses in cases of recruitment is due to the effect of the louder stimulus on the muscle reflex itself and not due to the timing of the neural energy leaving the cochlea.

Retrocochlear hearing losses.

Vestibulo-cochlear Schwannoma.   There are no published studies of the post-aural responses obtained in cases of eighth nerve Schwannoma but Gibson (1974) has tested three such cases. The responses in every case were small and the input-output functions did not indicate recruitment but whether such findings would occur in the atypical Schwannoma case displaying subjective recruitment is yet unknown.

Brainstem lesions.

Multiple sclerosis. Douek, Ashcroft and Humphries (1976) have reported that in many patients suffering from multiple sclerosis there is often a clear difference in the latency of the post-auricular responses obtained from the mastoid regions on each side of the head to monaural stimuli. Frequently the difference in latency exceeds 3 ms in these cases. It is possible that the post-aural response, using the 'crossed acoustic method', can provide a useful diagnostic tool for multiple sclerosis, although further work is needed. A similar observation has been noted using BER.

Gibson (1974) studied seven patients and found a similar delay in the response from one side of the head in five cases and also noted that the response configuration was often bizarre with complete unexplained absence of a response in three cases.

Brainstem tumours.   The post-aural responses, obtained using the 'crossed acoustic method', have been analysed in several patients with known brainstem tumours (Douek *et al.*, 1973; Gibson, 1974). All the proven cases that were tested showed some abnormality of the responses, usually the absence of either the ipsilateral or contralateral response. Because in the cases reported, the auditory and facial nerves were intact, these findings must be explained by another factor. It could be argued that this factor is merely the physiological unreliability of sonomotor responses. Indeed Cody and Bickford (1969) reported a normal subject in whom no response could be obtained from the contralateral mastoid on monaural stimulation; this may simply reflect on the use of a 1000 Hz stimulus with a slow onset rise time. Douek *et al.* (1973) appear to have evoked the response more reliably using a click stimulus and it would seem unlikely that such a large proportion of such a small group of patients would give abnormal responses unless it was due to a factor not present in the other subjects tested. Since all the subjects had proven brainstem lesions, it seems certain that, at least in some of the cases, the brainstem lesions had affected the responses.

The following is an analysis of the cases tested by Gibson (1974) with either brainstem tumours or disseminated sclerosis:

1. Absence of one contralateral (crossing) response—this was seen clearly in one patient with multiple sclerosis and may also have occurred in a second patient with carcinomatosis.

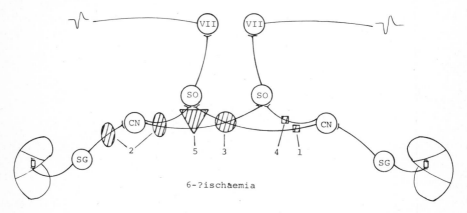

Fig. 6.18 A diagram of possible sites of disruption caused by lesions affecting the pathways of the post-auricular responses.

2. Absence of one contralateral response with a small or abnormal ipsilateral response—this abnormality was noted in one woman with a proven brainstem lesion affecting the region of the lower pons, one man with a large vestibular Schwannoma and two patients with carcinomatosis and known cerebral secondaries.

3. Absence of both contralateral responses—two patients with multiple sclerosis only gave post-aural responses from the mastoid behind the ear being stimulated.

4. Absence of one ipsilateral response—this was encountered in one man with multiple sclerosis, one patient with a haemorrhagic infarct of the cerebellum and in one patient with carcinomatosis with a known brainstem lesion.

5. Absence of both the ipsilateral and contralateral responses on stimulating one ear and the absence of the contralateral response on stimulating the other ear—this finding was noted in two patients with large brainstem tumours confirmed at autopsy soon after testing.

A speculative diagram to explain these findings is shown in Figure 6.18. It may be noted that lesions 1, 3 and 4 should only occur as a result of very localised brainstem damage and, in general, this was found to be the case. Lesions 2 and 5 should occur only with extensive destruction and most of the tumours produced this pattern of damage.

Several reports exist relating the absence of the contralateral intra-aural acoustic reflex to the presence of brainstem lesions (Greisen and Rasmussen, 1970; Steinberg and Lehnhart, 1974; Jerger et al., 1975). The post-auricular responses have an advantage over this method in that the responses can be obtained using stimulus intensities closer to the psycho-acoustic threshold thus enabling patients with partial hearing losses to be more easily tested. In many cases of non-recruiting hearing losses, the acoustic reflex cannot be elicited using the maximum output of the audiometer. The disadvantages of the post-aural response are its lack of reliability and the occurrence of false results. Precautions must always be taken to mask the opposite ear, to prevent cross-talk.

Whether the post-aural response can have any clinical value in detecting brainstem lesions remains doubtful. Unlike many of the tests used for diagnosis it is simple to apply and not at all unpleasant for the patient. It could provide a method of screening possible cases of brainstem involvement.

B.   The inion response

As a test of auditory acuity

Lowell et al. (1961) attempted to use the inion response as an indicator of hearing acuity in young children but found the response unsatisfactory. The main objection to the use of the inion response is that many workers have reported its presence on stimulating deaf ears and a possible vestibular excitation has been postulated.

As a means of neuro-otological diagnosis

No systematic studies of the inion response in pathological conditions have been published, although it may have some value in detecting lesions which interrupt the response pathway. A fascinating possibility is that the inion response may provide a measure of vestibular function, but studies attempting to relate its presence to the function of the semi-circular canals have been unrewarding. Townsend and Cody (1971) have suggested a link between this response and the saccule but again there is no published work which has explored the possibility.

Final remarks

The clinical use of sonomotor responses remains in doubt, although some interesting studies have been published regarding the post-auricular response.

7. The Contingent Negative Variation (CNV)

W.G. Walter working with his colleagues (1964) at Bristol, England, first reported the very slow potential changes known as the contingent negative variation (CNV). The CNV response appears as a slow DC shift in the baseline EEG activity following one stimulus as a result of conditioning a subject to expect a second stimulus to which he may be required to perform some task. The CNV is sometimes also known as the expectancy wave (E-wave). It reflects the difference in significance between the two separate stimuli and the intention of the subject to perform his task. Walter (1964) has suggested that the CNV is a shift of the apical cortical dendritic potentials in the direction of depolarisation to 'prime' the cortex for action, and that this reduction of the excitability threshold facilitates the ability of the cortex to respond, enhancing the efficiency of the overt activity.

Slow cerebral potential shifts were first reported in animals following the development of stable, high input impedance DC amplifiers. Caspers (1961) demonstrated a slow potential shift in rats which occurred in a negative direction in connection with locomotion, exploratory behaviour, alerting and orientating. Grooming, on the other hand, associated with a positive shift! He found the shift was not specific to any particular stimulus and was maximal in the central and frontal areas of the rat's brain. The shifts correlated with increased firing of the cells within the reticular formation and a negative steady potential shift altered to positive polarity when the rat became drowsy. He concluded that the steady potential gradient between the surface of the brain and the extracerebral reference electrode was generated by the apical dendritic network within the upper cortical layers of the brain.

Köhler and his colleagues (Köhler, Held and O'Connell, 1952; Köhler and O'Connell, 1957) demonstrated a slow potential shift that accompanied prolonged auditory and visual stimulation in cats, monkeys and humans. This DC perstimulatory shift has been examined further in humans by Keidel (1971a). They (Köhler et al., 1952) found the maximum negative shift to be at the vertex rather than, as they had expected, over the primary cortical areas. Later, Rowland (1961) reported slow potential shifts that occurred in cats after conditioning and were initially positive before becoming negative in polarity. They occurred during ten second intervals during which clicks signalled a forthcoming electric shock. The largest shifts were related to the earlier trials and the amplitude was related to the animal's drive to co-operate as it could be enhanced by food deprivation or feeding rewards (Rowland and Goldstone, 1963). A rather similar slow potential shift was reported by Wurtz (1966) which occurred in rats after electrical reinforcement following conditioning signals.

Another slow potential shift, first observed by Kornhuber and Deecke (1965), appears to be a readiness potential preceding voluntary movements and has its greatest amplitude over the contralateral Rolandic cortex. It is known as the 'Bereitschaftspotential' (BSP). McAdam and Searle (1969) have shown that an increase in motivation increases the amplitude of the BSP in a similar manner to the CNV. The BSP and CNV appear to be closely related except for the different scalp distributions and motivation.

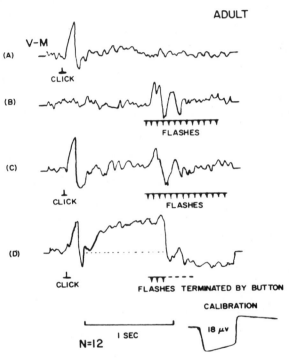

Fig. 7.1 The development of the CNV as a conditioned response (Cohen, J. (1969), by permission N.A.S.A.).

It was during this period of interest in slow potential shifts that Walter *et al*. (1964) gave their first important description of the CNV response in man. They described the basic paradigm for obtaining the CNV. This involves introducing first a *conditioning stimulus*, such as a pure tone, which is then followed by a second or *imperative stimulus*, for instance, a flash of light, to which the patient is asked to respond by performing a task, perhaps by pressing a button (the *operant response*). By repeating this paradigm several times, a conditioning process is established which is reminiscent of Pavlov's classic experiments. Eventually the subject begins to expect the arrival of the imperative stimulus and it is this expectancy which is related to the slow potential change known as the CNV (Fig. 7.1). An average of several trials are made, occurring at about four second intervals, so that the electrical response becomes clearly visible. The CNV can be used to estimate the pure tone audiometric threshold in patients by using a pure tone stimulus of a known intensity followed by a flash. Once clear CNV recordings are obtained, the intensity of the pure tone stimulus may be reduced and the patient will continue to yield a response until he can no longer hear the sound and so no longer expects the flash.

Much interest was aroused by the discovery of the CNV and soon several laboratories were investigating the response. Cohen and Walter (1966) demonstrated a CNV to an imperative stimulus consisting of pictures without the need for any physical operant response such as pressing a button. CNV responses have even been recorded with the subject merely required to 'think now' as the operant response. Irwin et al. (1966) and Cant and Bickford (1967) showed that the amplitude of the response increased together with the amount of effort required to press the bar as the operant response—the CNV amplitude was significantly greater when it was necessary to exert 14 pounds of pressure rather than 2 pounds of pressure. Large CNV amplitudes can often be associated with the degree of certainty with which the subject expects the oncoming imperative stimulus (Hillyard et al., 1971). Hillyard (1969) suggested that the amplitude of the CNV response might be correlated with the attention towards the imperative stimulus anticipated by the subject. McAdam (1966) had shown, however, that this factor was not related directly to CNV amplitude.

Chiorini (1966) demonstrated a CNV-like potential in cats during the acquisition of a conditioned avoidance response. Low and his co-workers (1966b) were able to demonstrate a CNV-like response in monkeys using a similar paradigm to humans.

Terminology

The term 'contingent negative variation' or 'CNV' is the most commonly used term to describe the negative slow potential shift discussed in this chapter. The term, CNV, was first coined by Walter et al. (1964) because the response, as first described, was contingent upon the occurrence of an imperative stimulus. Since then there have been a few objections to the term. Low et al. (1966a) objected as they could demonstrate that an imperative stimulus was not entirely necessary for the development of the response, so they used the term 'expectancy wave'. Nevertheless, the term 'CNV' has now become so firmly established that it is generally accepted.

Characteristics of the response

The distribution of the response

Walter (1964) initially believed that the CNV was derived mainly from the frontal areas of the brain and, in some subjects, swept backwards in time from the frontal pole, but this observation may have been influenced by the inclusion of potentials from eye movements (EAP). Later studies using monopolar and bipolar electrodes placed in various scalp positions showed that the CNV was centred near the vertex (Cohen, 1969; Vaughan, 1969) (Fig. 7.2—the electrodes are labelled in this figure as in other figures in this book according to the 10.20 international electrode system (Jasper, 1958)).

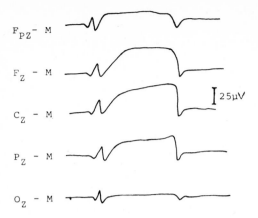

$F_{PZ} - M$

$F_Z - M$

$C_Z - M$ $\mathrm{I}\,25\mu V$

$P_Z - M$

$O_Z - M$

Fig. 7.2 The CNV as recorded from different scalp positions. (Key to positions as shown in Fig. 6.2).

Vaughan, Costa and Ritter (1968) have constructed isopotential maps of the CNV and found that it actually is derived from the region of the motor cortex. They have suggested that the CNV parallels an inhibition of on-going motor activity to set the stage for the expected release of a motor response. Cant and Bickford (1967) found that the topical distribution of the CNV altered under different test conditions. They reported that the presentation of a noxious stimulus following the operant response increased the amplitude of the CNV in the central and parietal regions, but when the subject was given the option of avoiding the noxious stimulus by making the operant response quickly within a set time limit, the CNV amplitude was increased mainly in the frontal region.

It may be concluded that the maximal CNV amplitude is usually obtained by using an active electrode placed near the vertex and that the reference electrode may be sited over the mastoid process. The amplitude of the response is reduced in frontal regions, further reduced in parietal areas and very small in occipital and posterior temporal positions.

The morphology of the response

The shape of the CNV response is specific to the individual subject, and also varies according to the experimental conditions. The commoner shapes of CNV responses are shown in Figure 7.3; among adults, approximately 40 per cent of

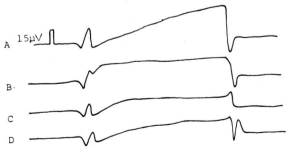

A $15\mu V$

B.

C

D

Fig. 7.3 Some of the commoner CNV patterns.

the responses are ramp-shaped, 33 per cent are rectangular and the remainder are atypically-shaped as in Figures 7.3C. and 7.3D. In some subjects the CNV may remain either for a short period after the imperative stimulus, or it may reduce briefly for about 0.1 sec. at the time of the imperative stimulus and then resume its negativity only gradually returning to the baseline after 1–2 seconds. This effect has been termed 'rebound' (Bostem *et al.*, 1967).

McAdam, Knott and Rebert (1969) have related the morphology of the CNV response to subjective certainty. They believed that when the subject was certain that the imperative stimulus would be delivered, the CNV was ramp-shaped, whereas if the subject was uncertain, a rectangular CNV response was more often obtained.

The relationship between CNV and CERA

A number of reports have attempted to relate the CNV to certain components of the slow cortical response (CERA). Bevan (1971) obtained CERA and CNV responses from 13 experienced divers exposed to increased air pressures simulating those of deep sea diving. Under conditions of increased pressure, the N_1 and P_2 CERA components were reduced in amplitude by approximately 60 per cent whilst no change in the amplitude of the CNV was observed. Bevan (1971) believed that this showed that the CNV and the N_1 and P_2 components of CERA were generated by different systems. He postulated that these CERA components were attenuated by passage through the ascending reticular system whilst the CNV involved the thalamic nuclei and was a self-propagating system generally independent of the reticular system.

Some work has been undertaken comparing the P_{300} component of CERA with the CNV response. In distinction to the other earlier components of CERA, the P_{300} component has a positive correlation to the subject's performance of tasks related to the stimulus. Donald and Goff (1971) presented subjects with a click which was followed two seconds later by a tone to which the subjects were asked to respond by pressing a button. During 75 per cent of the trials an unpleasant electric shock was given to the subject. When these electric shocks were related to pressing the button, the P_{300} amplitudes were increased, but no corresponding increase occurred in CNV amplitudes. The authors concluded that this experiment demonstrated that the process which increased the amplitude of the P_{300} was quite independent of the CNV.

The amplitude of the response

The average amplitude of the CNV response in adults is approximately $20\,\mu V$ (Walter, 1964; Low *et al.*, 1966a). The amplitudes vary considerably from subject and, in general, those subjects which give large amplitude CERA responses also give large amplitude CNV responses (Cohen, 1969). In adults, the mean amplitude of the CNV as recorded from the vertex is $21.4\,\mu V$ with a standard deviation of $4\,\mu V$ (Cohen, 1969). Low *et al.* (1966a) have reported CNV amplitudes as great as $50\,\mu V$ in subjects younger than 12 years of age. A few subjects do not give small responses and it is difficult to identify CNV responses of under $5\,\mu V$ in amplitude. The CNV is characteristically absent in psychopaths (Walter, 1966).

Factors affecting the amplitude.

The amplitude of the CNV is affected by fewer external test factors than other evoked potentials and the major factor appearing to affect it is the psychological state of the subject himself. The following test factors can affect the amplitude:

A. *Stimulus factors.* One fundamental difference between CNV audiometry and other methods of ERA is the requirement for two separate stimuli, the conditioning stimulus and the imperative stimulus. In the realm of audiometry, the conditioning stimulus is usually a pure tone burst. The characteristics of this stimulus are not critical and often a 300 ms tone burst with a gradual rise and decay are used as this allows good frequency specificity, but clicks and words may also be employed.

The nature of the imperative stimulus is not critical providing it can be perceived by the subject and usually a flash of light is used during CNV audiometry. If the subject is blind, an audible click may be used.

The operant task which makes the imperative stimulus significant, may effect the CNV amplitude, as it probably alters the degree of motivation of the subject. Certainly the CNV amplitude is increased when the subject has to perform a motor task such as pressing a button. Some of the factors have already been discussed in this chapter, for instance, the greater the effort required to complete the operant response, the larger the CNV potential.

B. *The inter-stimulus interval.* The time elapsing between the conditioning stimulus and the imperative stimulus is important. McAdam, Knott and Rebert (1969) found that CNV amplitudes were significantly larger if the interval between these stimuli was between 0.8 and 1.6 seconds. If this interval is divided into quarters then, for the same subject, the relative growth of amplitude for each quarter is usually similar. The point of time at which the response reaches its maximum may depend on the timing of the operant response (Cohen, 1969).

C. *Amplitudes during the whole testing period.* The acquisition, maintenance and extinction of the CNV has attracted attention. McAdam *et al.* (1969) showed that the amplitude of the CNV develops to its maximum during the acquisition trial and later decreases during the practice trials. Walter *et al.* (1964) suggested that the CNV response could be maintained indefinitely providing the subject retained interest, and that this interest was best maintained by having the subject perform an operant response. Certainly the CNV develops more quickly (within a few trials) when an interesting operant task is required (Low *et al.*, 1966a).

When the subject is not warned, the CNV disappears progressively over approximately 30 trials once the imperative stimulus is omitted (Walter *et al.*, 1964). On warning the subject, Walter *et al.* (1964) reported that the CNV was extinguished immediately when the imperative stimulus ceased, but Low *et al.* (1966a) found that often it disappeared more slowly over 6–12 trials.

When an imperative stimulus follows the conditioning stimulus no more than 40–45 per cent of the time, the CNV amplitude is reduced (Walter *et al.*, 1964). The CNV can still be obtained in patients of high intelligence when reinforcement by an imperative stimulus only occurs in 30 per cent of trials. Walter (1966) has suggested that, when the CNV persists when the probability of reinforcement is low, the subjects are seekers of stress, and when the CNV cannot be obtained even with a high probability of reinforcement, the subjects are anxious and neurotic.

The latency of the response

The latency of the onset of the CNV potential is difficult to measure since it develops amongst potentials which are late components of the evoked potential to the conditioning stimulus. Rebert and Knott (1970) found that the CNV did not commence until at least 400 ms had elapsed following the presentation of the conditioning stimulus. They suggested an average onset latency of 467 ms. The latency of the maximum amplitude of the response is variable and usually lies within 450–900 ms.

Exclusion of possible contaminating potentials

The motor 'intention' potential or Bereitschaftspotential (BSP).   This potential, described earlier in this chapter, occurs in humans as a slow potential shift that precedes a voluntary muscle movement by approximately half a second. The BSP is inconsistent in nature and has its maximum amplitude over the contralateral motor cortex. It has been shown that the CNV response is not identical with the BSP since the CNV may be obtained using an operant response which does not involve a muscular movement. Nevertheless the BSP and CNV are evidently closely related and without doubt the BSP contributes to the amplitude of the CNV recorded in some circumstances.

Eye artefact potentials.   There are several ways in which the movements of the eyes can produce electrical potentials but the main source results from a change in the axis of the eye which alters the corneoretinal potential or electro-oculogram (EOG). This potential is familiar to clinicians as it is used in electronystagmography. The potential may be carried by volume conduction to electrodes placed on the scalp. Hillyard (1974) lists the other less direct ways in which eye movements may produce electrical artefacts, and he mentions details of methods of recognising and eliminating eye artefact potentials.

It is certain that eye movements alone do not account for the CNV potential. Compelling evidence lies in two fields:

1.   The CNV is similar whether obtained from electrodes placed on the surface of the scalp or from electrodes placed directly on the exposed cortex and well away from the frontal areas (Walter *et al.*, 1964).

2.   A CNV-like response can be recorded from animals after their eyes have been removed (Chiorini, 1969). Human evidence has been gathered from subjects with glass eyes (Low *et al.*, 1966a), for in these subjects no corneoretinal potential can exist but the CNV is present.

Although it is clear that the CNV exists as a separate potential to the EOG, it seems certain that in some circumstances EOG is superimposed on to CNV recordings. The most extensive work on this subject has been undertaken by Hillyard (Hillyard and Galambos, 1970; Hillyard, 1974). He described the CNV as being composed of two potentials, the 'true' CNV (tCNV) and the 'eye artefact potential' (EAP) which is derived from EOG. He compared computer-averaged

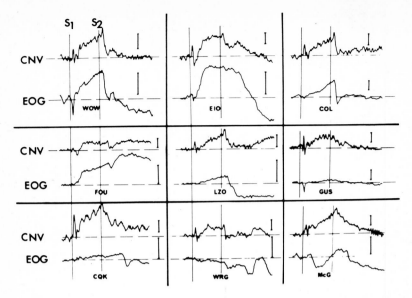

Fig. 7.4 Typical computer-averaged NCV (Cz channel) and simultaneously recorded EOG deflections from nine subjects, during eight S1–S2 response trials with eyes closed. Calibration pulse, Cz channel 20 μV; EOG 100 μV (Hillyard, S.A. & Galambos, R. (1970), by permission *Electroencephalography and Clinical Neurophysiology*).

tracings of the CNV, derived from mastoid and vertex electrodes, with a simultaneously obtained transorbital EOG recording obtained from electrodes placed above and below one eye (Fig 7.4). By such a procedure, he found that 23 per cent of CNV recordings, in average subjects, were composed of a negative EAP because of a tendency for the subjects to move their eyes downwards in synchrony with the CNV. As a result, most workers now recommend that CNV recordings are obtained with the eyes open and optically-fixated.

The test and test/retest reliability

The test reliability of CNV is fair because the response does diminish as the subject gets accustomed to the proceedure and as the effect of conditioning wanes. Moreover, the CNV cannot be identified in 10 per cent of normal subjects (Walter, 1964b; Burian, Gestring and Haider, 1969). The possibility of encountering a non-responsive subject cannot be overlooked. This possibility is greater in young children, psychopaths and anxious or neurotic subjects. Prevec, Lokar and Cernelc (1974) tested eight normal adults and obtained CNV at 5–10 dB SL in every case. The CNV was most apparent at near threshold levels.

The test/retest reliability is fair. Subjects with clear CNV on one occasion tend to continue to give a good response at later test sessions. The repeated testing of subjects who do not have identifiable CNV does reduce the number of non-responders to about three per cent (Prevec *et al.*, 1974).

Instrumentation

The apparatus typically used for CNV audiometry is shown in Figure 7.5.

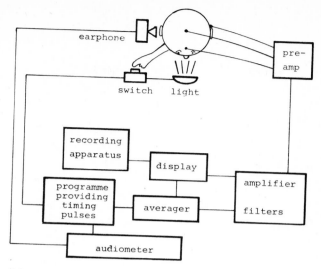

Fig. 7.5 A block diagram of the typical apparatus for CNV audiometry.

Most of the equipment is similar to that described in Chapter Two, so this account is restricted to the specific requirements for CNV audiometry.

The test environment

Ideally the subject should be tested in a sound-proof chamber, and is generally seated comfortably with the neck supported. The chamber also contains the pre-amplifiers into which the electrode leads are inserted, close to the subject's head; the earphones or loudspeaker, a switch for the operant response and a light, directly in front of the subject, giving the imperative stimulus.

The stimulus generation

Two separate stimuli must be provided and each must receive a trigger pulse which is time-locked to the analysis sweep. The first is the conditioning stimulus which occurs after a short pre-stimulus analysis delay of 0.5–1.5 sec. This, in the case of auditory work, is a pure tone burst and its shape is comparatively unimportant; generally a 300 ms tone burst with a slow rise and decay time is used to allow good frequency specificity. Clicks and words may also be used. The second stimulus, or imperative stimulus, is generally a weak flash of light lasting 0.5 sec which occurs between 0.8 and 1.6 sec after the conditioning stimulus. Larger CNV responses are obtained when there is a provision for the light to be extinguished by making an operant response (pressing a button).

The conditioning stimulus may be of any frequency which is audible to the subject. The intensity of the stimulus is varied in 10 or 5 dB steps so that the threshold intensity can be determined, the absence of a CNV response indicating, in most cases, the subject's psychophysical hearing threshold. Masking facilities may be needed.

The recording apparatus

Electrodes. Reliable, non-polarising electrodes are essential for recording

CNV. Hillyard (1974) recommends the use of commercially-available silver/silver chloride pellets enclosed in plastic housing. Standard silver/silver chloride EEG dome-shaped electrodes may also be used and it helps to keep pairs shorted together. The electrodes must have a good coating of silver chloride to help avoid polarisation. The skin to electrode resistance should be kept to a minimum and should be lower than 3 kΩ. Badly applied electrodes with high and widely differing resistances are a common cause of difficulty and interference. With experience, these troubles are more easily detected and overcome. A device to measure the resistance between electrodes is an advantage. A resistance meter and a battery may cause problems in CNV work as it may polarise the electrodes. An AC method of measuring the electrode impedance, is a distinct advantage.

Amplifiers.   The amplifiers must be DC coupled and built to low noise biological specifications. The total gain required as in the order of 10^5.

Filter settings (bandpass).   Some of the unwanted electrical noise can be excluded by frequency filtering. The high pass filter has to be either DC or an extremely low frequency. Hillyard (1974) reports that the advantages of DC amplification outweigh the minor inconveniences, as it yields a wholly undistorted CNV waveform. He finds that the alternative AC recording with a long time constant (10 seconds approximates a bandpass of 0.16 Hz) will distort a monophasic negative waveform into a negative-positive ensemble. Many workers, however, do not have the apparatus for DC amplification and in these circumstances a filter setting of 0.016 Hz is suitable for testing adults, although if children are to be tested, there can still be problems with DC artefacts caused by movement and a high pass filter setting of 0.16–0.32 Hz may produce better results. The low pass filter setting is often chosen between 12–16 Hz, as this conveniently excludes the mains power frequency.

The averager.   A small computer or a purpose-built averager may be used. The CNV is best observed when only a few epochs or trials are averaged (Walter *et al.*, 1965); usually 10–30 are sufficient. The analysis time should be arranged so that a short period of the on-going activity is included, as this provides the baseline for measuring the response. A typical analysis period is of four seconds duration. It consists, typically, of a period of 1.2 seconds before the presentation of the conditioning stimulus (pre-analysis period), 300 ms during which the pure tone conditioning stimulus is delivered, 1.0 seconds between the conditioning stimulus and the imperative stimulus and after which a further 1.5 seconds of analysis. The imperative stimulus is usually of an indeterminate period, as it is terminated by the subject making the operant response. The interval between each period of analysis may be varied but usually lies between 2–5 seconds.

The monitor oscilloscope.   Because only a few trials are averaged, artefacts can easily lead to misinterpretation if unwittingly included into the averaged response recording. A careful watch should be made of the on-going electrical activity so that any sudden changes can be noted. Eye movements may produce DC potentials which can easily be mistaken for CNV responses.

Permanent recording of results and analysis
    CNV testing is a prolonged procedure and most workers find it advantageous

to record all the data on a FM magnetic tape recorder and analyse it off-line. The experts in this field programme computers to identify trials containing artefacts so that these can be excluded from the averaged response (Rousseau, Bostem and Dongier, 1968). With tape-recorded data, the CNV can be constructed using different trials, in a cross-cutting fashion, allowing the significance of each response to be determined.

Testing procedures

The subject must be awake and attentive. Movements of the head and neck must be limited to prevent the generation of electrical artefacts. The subject is therefore seated comfortably with the neck supported. To minimise eye movement potentials (EAP), the subject is asked to keep his gaze fixed on the light bulb which provides the operant response.

Electrodes. Before applying the electrodes it is essential that all traces of grease are removed from the underlying skin (e.g. using acetone). Secure contact between electrode and skin is essential to prevent extensive baseline drifting during averaging. Electrode lead sway must also be avoided. Picton and Hillyard (1972) report that the baseline potential can be greatly stabilised by puncturing the skin under each electrode with a sterile needle, as this attenuates electrodermal variations.

Newly-applied electrodes generally cause drifting for several minutes as the interfaces gradually reach an electrochemical equilibrium. It is advisable to wait for 10–15 minutes after applying electrodes before beginning the testing.

If the baseline drifts less than $15-20\,\mu V$ per minute, satisfactory CNV recordings can be made. Bad drifting is usually due to a poorly applied electrode which has to be identified and replaced. Occasionally, the cause of drifting cannot be found, but even so, measured CNV amplitudes can usually be corrected to compensate for this factor.

The basic electrode positions are; active electrode on the vertex, reference electrode over either mastoid process and earth electrode on the forehead. Hillyard (1974), however, advises a minimum array consisting of a row of three or four electrodes along the mid-line from occiput to frontal scalp to measure the anterior-posterior gradient of the CNV, with an earlobe or a mastoid reference site. He also advises recording the electro-oculogram (EOG) and the galvanic skin potential from the palm to provide further information to exclude possible artefact sources. This array is probably beyond the scope of the equipment available in all but the most sophisticated centres.

Subject's instructions. The subject has to be told the relevance of the various stimuli and instructed as to when he is to make the operant response. He is told that he will hear a pure tone signal, which may be extremely faint, and this will warn him that the light is about to flash on. He is asked to extinguish the light by pressing a button as quickly as possible. Obviously these instructions vary according to the particular test to be performed.

Clinical use of CNV

There are no reports that the CNV has yet been used as a routine clinical test, but several studies have been undertaken which examine the clinical potential of the response. The possible uses of CNV for auditory threshold estimation and for neuro-otological diagnosis are discussed.

As a method of estimating the auditory threshold

The advantage of CNV as a means of objective audiometry is that, unlike other methods of ERA, it does show that the stimulus has actually been perceived. It offers a direct audiometric measure. There are, however, many disadvantages. Not the least is that, to obtain a clear response, an operant response is required such as the pressing of a button. Sceptics might add that more information can be gained regarding the auditory threshold by merely observing whether or not the subject presses the button, making it unnecessary to analyse the EEG and saving the need for expensive equipment. CNV audiometry is hardly practical in young children in its present form. Young children do not often develop CNV potentials (Walter, 1966) and the need for an operant response, passive co-operation throughout the session and the avoidance of sedatives make the management of the disturbed child impossible. Prevec, Ribaric and Butinar (1977) have suggested that better results are obtained when testing pre-scool children on using a cartoon as the imperative stimulus. Using this type of stimulus, they recorded CNV in 9/9 children within ±7.5dB of their psycho-acoustic threshold.

Pure tone audiometry.   Prevec, Lokar and Cernelc (1974) evaluated the use of CNV for the estimation of the pure tone auditory threshold of adults. They report that 10 per cent of normal, healthy subjects fail to develop a recordable CNV. In contrast to the findings with other methods of ERA, the amplitude of the response does not decrease as the stimulus intensity is diminished (Prevec *et al.*, 1974; Rapin *et al.*, 1966). The CNV, in fact, is often larger when the stimulus is near the threshold of perception (Prevec *et al.*, 1974; Rebert *et al.*, 1967). This may be due to an increase in the concentration of the subject when he can barely hear the warning sound.

Speech audiometry.   Burian and his co-workers (Burian, Gestring and Haider, 1969; Burian *et al.*, 1972) have used CNV as a method of objective speech audiometry. They have named this use of CNV as 'language electric response audiometry' (LERA). The subject is conditioned in such a way that he associates only meaningful words with the presentation of the imperative light stimulus and not the meaningless words which may also be presented. They tested two adult patients with aphasia (Burian *et al.*, 1972). One patient, aged 46 years, was severely aphasic following a neurosurgical removel of an astrocytoma. Soon after the operation, no difference in the CNV response to meaningful or meaningless words could be demonstrated, but several months later, after he had recovered, he was able to discriminate and only developed a CNV response to the meaningful words. Obviously it would be fascinating if such a test could be applied to children but unfortunately the practical difficulties are immense.

As a means of neuro-otological diagnosis

The CNV could provide a fascinating diagnostic tool for psychiatrists and psychologists who are concerned with higher cortical functions. It does not offer so much of interest to workers interested in the functioning of the lower parts of the auditory tract. Most of this topic has been discussed previously in this chapter. Psychopathic subjects have great difficulty in establishing a CNV Conflicting reports have been published regarding CNV amplitudes in patients with anxiety neuroses. Knott and Irwin (1968) found smaller amplitudes in patients with manifest anxiety states, whilst Low and his colleagues (1967) found no such correlation. Walter (1967) has reported that in intelligent patients, the CNV can be maintained even when the imperative stimulus only follows 30 per cent of the conditioning stimuli, whereas, in patients of lesser intelligence and those that are 'seekers of stress' the CNV cannot be obtained unless the probability of reinforcement is high.

Final remarks

The CNV has not yet been introduced into clinical use and it does have several disadvantages as a method of ERA, so the discussion in this book regarding CNV has been kept brief. There is, however, a potential application for CNV as a means of assessing higher cortical functions. The use of CNV in determining whether a word has truly been understood or is meaningless has interesting possibilities. For instance, it could be used in counter-espionage to reveal whether or not the subject has an understanding of a foreign language. More sinister applications could involve presenting pleasant and unpleasant conditioning stimuli and then, for example, determining whether the male subject is homosexual by presenting a picture of a naked man. Obviously such applications are highly speculative and would involve variables such as co-operation and response reliability. Perhaps this is as well, for it could provide the means for an unwelcome (and unethical) intrusion into the privacy of the human mind.

8. The Middle Latency (Early Cortical) Responses

When Geisler and his colleagues (1958) first averaged the electrical responses obtained from scalp electrodes using click stimuli, they discovered several potentials with onset latencies varying from 8 ms to 30 ms. Initially, these potentials were thought to be neurogenic in origin but later the studies of Bickford and his group (1963a, 1963b) offered irrefutable evidence of myogenic contamination. It is now accepted that the acoustically-evoked responses (latencies 8–40 ms) derived from placing the active, or monopolar, electrode directly over the post-aural region or over the inion are almost entirely myogenic (*see* Chapter Six). There is good evidence, however, that at least some of the middle latency responses (8–60 ms) obtained using electrodes placed near the parietal region of the scalp are neurogenic.

Mast (1963, 1965) studied the responses recorded from parietal and vertex (Pl, Cz) electrode placements. He found that the parietal response differed from the inion sonomotor response in that it was recordable under conditions of both forward and backward neck traction, it was detectable using low stimulus intensities, it was stable in pattern, it had a long recovery period and it did not increase exponentially in response amplitude with increasing stimulus intensity. He concluded that the potentials which constitute the parietal response probably contain both myogenic and neurogenic components. Other workers have supported this theory of a dual origin (Borsanyi and Blanchard, 1964; Lowell, 1965; Goldstein, 1965; Vaughan and Ritter, 1970). A convincing supportive study was undertaken by Ruhm, Walker and Flanigin (1967). These workers compared the scalp recordings, in the same two subjects, with recordings taken directly from the surface of the brain during surgery. The response components were similar in latency under the two conditions but the amplitude of the responses was three times greater when recordings were taken directly from the cortex. More recently, Skinner and Shimota (1974) have provided further evidence of a neurogenic component by demonstrating that significant binaural interaction takes place during the formation of these middle latency responses.

Picton *et al*. (1974) suggested that the neurogenic components of the middle latency responses were derived from the 'auditory areas of the thalamus' and the primary auditory cortex, but found that these neurogenic components were easily obscured by myogenic activity. Davis (1976) concluded also 'the distinction between neurogenic and myogenic (sonomotor) components is not complete. The latter are often present, even at low sensation levels (personal observation), and the strong possibility exists that they may sometimes be out of phase with, and therefore cancel, the neurogenic components.'.

Terminology

Mast (1963, 1965) originally named the series of evoked potentials with onset latencies of less than 60 ms, 'the short latency responses'. Other contemporary workers have used the terms 'fast or early responses'. Any of these terms were suitable at the time, as they conveniently separated the responses from the 'slow cortical responses' (CERA) and the 'very slow cortical responses' (CNV). With the more recent introduction of 'very fast responses' (ECochG and BER), the 8–60 ms responses have become known as the 'middle latency responses'. The current use of the term 'middle latency responses' is associated almost exclusively with neurogenic components rather than sonomotor components. To stress this distinction, the middle latency responses are sometimes referred to as 'the early cortical response', but it should be remembered that the earlier components are probably thalamic in origin and the exclusion of all myogenic elements is unlikely. Perhaps Davis (1971) was wise in stating that the only certain method of describing a response is to name the polarity and latency of each of the constituent peaks. It is apt, therefore, to consider at this time the configuration of the middle latency responses.

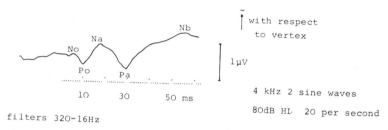

Fig. 8.1 The waveform of the middle latency responses.

Response configuration

The waveform of the middle latency responses is still somewhat uncertain, as different investigators have used recording systems with filters set at different cut-off frequencies (Lane, Mendel and Kupperman, 1974). The effect of altering the bandpass is discussed in further detail later in this chapter but it should be noted at this point that lowering the frequency of the low pass filter results in a prolongation of the peak latencies.

The waveform of the response is described as consisting of two major positive peaks (vertex referred to mastoid) and three major negative peaks. The peaks have been labelled No, Po, Na, Pa, and Nb (Goldstein and Rodman, 1967) to avoid confusion with the symbols N1, P1, N2, P2 etc. which are used to describe the slow cortical response. It may sometimes be possible to identify a sixth peak, Pb. Typical responses are shown in Figure 8.1.

The peak latencies of the responses usually occur within the following limits depending on the bandpass of the system used: No 8–10 ms, Po 10–13 ms, Na 16–30 ms, Pa 30–45 ms, Nb 40–60 ms and Pb 55–80 ms. The latency of the responses is quite consistent within the same subject and Pa is, perhaps, the most stable of the individual peaks. The peak-to-peak amplitudes vary from about 0.7 to 3.0 μV with the largest peak being Nb. Goldstein and Rodman (1967) found that the combination of Na and Pa provided the best means of identifying the responses. The No and Pb peaks are not always identifiable. The No response is probably identical with the Jewett V wave recorded as part of BER, so its loss of reliability is likely to be due to the narrowing of the recording bandpass limits. The Nb and Pb peaks may well be synonymous with the early components of the slow cortical response. A worrying feature of the 'neurogenic' middle latency responses is that their early waveform overlaps closely with the waveform of the post-auricular sonomotor response (Chapter Six).

Some characteristics of the responses

Electrode positions and the bilateral nature of the responses

Electrodes placed on or around the parietal region of the scalp provide the clearest responses (Mast, 1965; Vaughan and Ritter, 1970). The responses are usually recorded using a vertex electrode, referred either to a mastoid or an earlobe electrode with the earth electrode placed on a convenient site such as the forehead.

When Chatrian, Petersen and Lazarte (1960) placed electrodes directly on the surgically-exposed cortex, they reported that the middle latency responses showed a marked predominance on the contralateral hemisphere to the side of the stimulated ear. Sem-Jacobsen *et al.* (1956) found that binaural stimulation resulted in larger responses than monaural stimulation. It is surprising, therefore, that Peters and Mendel (1974) found that the configuration (peak latencies and amplitudes) of the scalp-recorded responses was essentially unaltered regardless of whether one ear, the other ear or both ears were stimulated. Provided this latter study is confirmed, it would appear that it is only necessary to place electrodes on one side of the head for threshold determination procedures.

Effect of changes in muscle tone

It is known that sonomotor responses, such as the inion response and the post-aural response, show marked variations with changes in muscle tone. Mast (1965) reported that the parietal middle latency responses were not altered by head movements. Harker *et al.* (1977), testing a normally-hearing volunteer at 50 dB SL, found that the responses were not altered by the administration of the drug succinycholine (Scoline ®) which produced total muscle paralysis. They also noted that the waveform was unaltered by diazepam (Valium ®) sedation. This evidence indicates that the middle latency responses are not entirely sonomotor and is suggestive of a neural origin.

Effect of subject state

Sem-Jacobsen *et al.* (1965), using cortically-placed electrodes, found that the amplitude of the responses decreased with increasing depth of anaesthesia and noted that no responses could be obtained in deep sleep. Mendel and Goldstein (1969), however, have shown that no gross alteration of the scalp-recorded responses occurs with the subject sitting in darkness, sitting in the light or sitting reading. These workers (Mendel and Goldstein, 1971; Mendel, 1974a), in fact, first noted that scalp-recorded middle latency responses were stable in sleep; the latency was not affected by deep sleep but the amplitude of the waveform was slightly reduced. They found that the REM stage of sleep was the most conducive to good recordings. Kupperman and Mendel (1974) have recently reported that the responses are stable even when the sleep is induced artificially with secobarbital. This stability of the middle latency responses in sleep is important, especially as the test is often directed towards assessing the hearing status of a paediatric population, the members of which are not often willing to sit still for long periods.

The effects of stress have also been reported. Hypoxia, hyperventilation and body acceleration through space all have the effects of increasing the latencies and of reducing the amplitudes of the response components (Freeman, 1965). During these periods of stress, no concomitant effect was noticed to occur in the ongoing EEG records.

Effect of stimulus conditions

Stimulus duration.   The effects of stimulus duration have been studied by Skinner and Antinoro (1971). They reported no consistent changes on using stimulus durations which varied from 1.5 to 4.0 ms. Kupperman (1970) reported similar findings.

Stimulus rise time.   All the reports on the effect of stimulus rise times note that the faster rise times yield larger and more consistent responses. Lane and Kupperman (1969) have noted that the amplitude of the responses is greater when it is elicited by clicks rather than by pure tone stimuli. Zerlin, Naunton and Mowry (1973) have used third octave clicks in an attempt to obtain some frequency specificity, as they too found that low frequency pure tone bursts evoked the responses inadequately. Skinner and Antinoro (1971) have elicited responses using a wide range of stimulus rise times. They found that rise times greater than 25 ms would not often produce identifiable responses, whilst stimuli with a rise time of 10 μs (presumably they had the use of an excellent transducer), always resulted in clear responses. Kupperman and Mendel (1974), in a sleep study, compared the response threshold obtained using tone pip stimuli and clicks with the auditory threshold. They reported that responses could be identified at 20 dB SL using a 500 Hz stimulus and at 10 dB SL using 1 kHz, 4 kHz and click stimuli (group mean data). Similar reports all showing the need for a fast stimulus rise time to elicit the responses have been published by Kupperman (1970), Beiter and Hogan (1973) and other workers.

The requirement for the middle latency responses for a 'rapid-rise' stimulus is a disadvantage shared with ECochG, BER and the sonomotor responses.

Stimulus decay time.   Most reports have shown that the timing of the stimulus decay is relatively unimportant. Responses are effectively produced only by the onset of the stimulus, i.e., they are on-responses (Hood, 1974).

Effect of prolonged or repeated stimulation

The middle latency responses are reputed to show no evidence of fatigue or habituation even during prolonged or repeated bouts of stimulation. Mendel and Goldstein (1971) reported no habituation of the responses obtained from one sleeping subject even after presenting 250 000 clicks.

Effect of stimulus repetition rate

The middle latency responses tolerate much faster stimulus repetition rates than the slow cortical responses. Mendel (1974) advises a stimulus repetition rate of 6–10 per second. Unfortunately, no detailed study of the effect of changing the interstimulus interval is available.

Effect of stimulus frequency

Kupperman (1970) has shown that the waveform of the middle responses is not as dependent on the frequency of the stimulus as on the stimulus rise time. His study employed only audible frequencies.

Effect of altering the stimulus intensity

Amplitude and intensity functions.   Madell and Goldstein (1972) have plotted the mean peak-to-peak amplitudes of 24 normally-hearing young adults using click stimuli presented at a rate of 9.6 per second (Fig. 8.2). It was noted that not all the subjects showed a consistent relationship between stimulus intensity and response amplitude. It was found, however, that the amplitude/intensity functions of the middle latency responses were quite different from those reported for sonomotor responses. Madell and Goldstein (1972) were unable to demonstrate any correlation between loudness magnitude judgements and the amplitudes of any components of the responses.

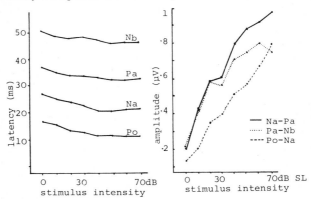

Fig. 8.2 The latency/intensity (left) and the amplitude/intensity (right) functions of the components of the middle latency responses (Adapted from Madell and Goldstein (1972)).

Latency and intensity functions.   The relationship between the latency of each of the peaks and the stimulus intensity was also described by Madell and Goldstein (1972) (Fig. 8.2). The latency/intensity functions show a similarity to those of the post-aural sonomotor response.

Effect of altering bandwidth recording limits

The use of 'filtering' is an effective means of excluding unwanted electrical activity from the response in ERA but it must be remembered that filtering alters

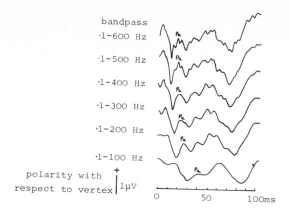

Fig. 8.3 The alteration of the waveform resulting from limiting the bandpass of the recording system (Adapted from Lane *et al.* (1974)).

the waveform. Lane *et al.* (1974) have shown the effect on the middle latency responses of altering the bandwidth of the recording system (Fig. 8.3). An alteration in both the amplitudes and the latencies of the peaks occurred. The amplitude distortion is a desired result of filtering, as it makes the presence or absence of responses much easier to judge. Phase distortion serves no beneficial purpose and it causes quite marked shifts in the latencies of the peaks in the waveform. Shifts in peak latencies of the middle responses occur chiefly on reducing the level of the low pass filter and probably account for the different waveforms reported by different workers.

The sensory receptor of the middle latency responses

It is not known yet whether the middle latency responses can only be generated by stimulation of the cochlea or whether they may be mediated through other sensory receptors such as tactile or vestibular receptors. Perhaps some caution should be exercised in the interpretation of small responses to high intensities of stimulation until this important question is answered.

The test and test/retest reliability

Hood (1974) states that the middle latency responses are stable, easy to elicit and bear a close relationship to the auditory threshold, but this view is not shared by all workers. The responses are of small amplitude and may easily become buried in the on-going EEG and random myogenic activity. Lane, Kupperman and Goldstein (1971) were unable to identify the responses in four out of ten young normally-hearing adults using 1 kHz 50 dB SL stimuli. They observed responses, however, in all ten subjects using click stimuli.

Madell and Goldstein (1972) reported that most subjects gave reproducible response waveforms when testing was performed on separate occasions after an interval of two days. Some subjects, however, did show considerable differences. Unfortunately they did not quantify this statement.

It would appear that the middle latency responses in a small number of subjects are unreliable and, in this respect, they parallel the post-aural sonomotor responses. The problem of possible 'non-responders' hampers their use in assessing the auditory threshold, especially in the lower frequency range.

The relationship to the (psychophysical) auditory threshold

Goldstein and Rodman (1967) investigated the relationship between the middle latency responses click threshold and the auditory threshold to the same stimuli. It may be seen (Table 1) that positive responses were identified in 80 per cent of the subjects at 30 dB SL and in about half the subjects at ± 5 dB SL. Ten per cent of the control trials were falsely judged to have yielded positive responses. At −5 dB SL, 55 per cent of the subjects were thought to have given positive responses, implying that either this test is more sensitive than the psycho-physical threshold or that false positive responses are very common at close-to-threshold levels. Interestingly, Horowitz, Larson and Sances (1966) had reported finding more difficulty in identifying responses close to the auditory threshold level in normally-hearing subjects than in patients with partial hearing losses.

The relationship between the responses threshold and the auditory threshold in sleep was reported by Kupperman and Mendel (1974). The mean difference between auditory threshold and the level at which the two 'judges' believed the responses present (yes-decisions) for 50 per cent of the trials was reported as 10 dB SL for 1 kHz and 4 kHz tone pips and click stimuli.

It would appear that the identification of the responses threshold does require a degree of skill. It could be said that this is rather a 'subjective' form of 'objective' audiometry.

dB SL	Na + Pa + Nb		Na + Pa		Pa + Nb	
	N	%	N	%	N	%
60	10	50	17	85	10	50
30	9	45	18	90	9	45
10	8	40	16	80	8	40
5	8	40	14	70	9	45
0	6	30	10	50	8	40
−5	2	10	11	55	2	10
−10	1	5	5	25	1	5
silent control	0	0	1	5	0	0
silent control	2	10	4	20	3	15

Table 1. Subjects (total N = 20) meeting the latency criteria for a positive response: Na, 16.25–30.00 ms; Pa, 30.00–45.00 ms; Nb, 46.25–56.25 ms. (Goldstein, R. & Rodman, L.B. (1967)).

Frequency specificity of the responses

There is an inescapable dilemma in that only a stimulus with a fast rise time evokes responses reliably and yet such a stimulus is not precise in frequency, especially below 1 kHz. Some compromise must be made and most workers have favoured the use of a tone pip (Kupperman and Mendel, 1974, *inter alia*). Zerlin, Naunton and Mowry (1973) have used third octave clicks and believed that they could reliably evoke responses that were frequency specific even at 500 Hz. The recent work on the frequency specificity of the stimuli used for electrocochleography (see Chapter Four) suggests that tone pips are only frequency specific at low intensities (0–40 dB HL).

Instrumentation

The apparatus required for the middle latency responses is very similar to that needed for other methods of ERA and the basic details are described in Chapter Two. The specific requirements are listed in the following paragraphs.

The test environment

It is an advantage to perform the testing in a chamber which is electrically-screened especially from mains power sources because the response is small and easily obscured by such activity. It is also advantageous, but not so essential, to have a sound-proofed test chamber. The subjects must be tested while they are relaxed, otherwise the response is obscured by myogenic activity. Most workers ask the subject to lie on a couch or to sit in a chair with the head well supported. Because young children are usually sedated, some means of keeping them under constant observation during testing is essential.

The stimulus requirements

Stimulus envelope. As previously mentioned the optimum stimulus is a click with a sharp rise time ($10\,\mu s$–$100\,\mu s$) but such a stimulus is not very frequency specific. Tone bursts with sharp onsets may also be used. Zerlin *et al.* (1973) have suggested third octave clicks. Mendel (1974) recommends a stimulus envelope of 2 ms rise time, 2 ms plateau and 2 ms decay time, as such an envelope can be used to obtain a reasonable indication of the cochlear function within the range of frequency between 500 Hz and 8 kHz.

Stimulus repetition rate. The most commonly used stimulus repetition rate is 10 per second. In Goldstein's laboratory, at the University of Wisconsin, a rate of 9.6 per second is employed, as this rate has the advantage of being out of phase with the mains power frequencies. 1000 or more stimuli are needed in each epoch to recover the responses from the background electrical activity. It takes, therefore, approximately two minutes to obtain each averaged waveform.

Stimulus transducer. A good quality transducer is needed to provide an acoustic waveform that is free of click artefacts. Most adult subjects are tested using earphones and these also can be attached to the sleeping child.

Stimulus calibration. The brief stimuli used are difficult to calibrate with accuracy. Several methods are discussed in Chapter Two although none is entirely satisfactory. The stimuli are usually delivered in 10 dB increments to a maximum of 110 or 120 dB HL.

The recording equipment

Electrodes. The responses may be obtained using standard EEG disc electrodes similar to those advocated for CERA. Many workers use silver/silver chloride dome-shaped electrodes. These should be well-coated with silver chloride to help prevent polarization.

Amplifiers. Low noise biological amplifiers are essential. The total gain required to visualise the response is in the order of 10^5.

Filter settings (bandpass). Although filtering of unwanted electrical activity is essential to allow responses to be easily identified, such filtering does lead to amplitude reduction and some phase distortion. Obviously a compromise has to be made. Mendel (1974b) recommends a bandpass between 25 Hz and 175 Hz with a 'roll-off' of 6 dB per octave.

The averager.   Any small purpose-built averager will suffice. Goldstein and his colleagues use a Fabri-Tek 1052S signal averager. The analysis window is usually in the order of 100 ms and approximately 10 memory points are required for each millisecond of analysis.

The monitor oscilloscope.   It is important to have a means available of monitoring the background electrical activity as large extraneous potentials can easily swamp the response. A practised observer can recognise such fluctuations and avoid the error of mistaking a sudden change for positive response.

The FM tape recorder.   It is important to be able to analyse the responses retrospectively. If the data are recorded on a tape recorder, they can be analysed at leisure. It helps considerably, when the responses are used to predict audiometric threshold, to be able to exclude sections of the tape which include high levels of background electrical noise from the averaged waveform. Recordings also provide the opportunity for a second observer to analyse the averaging process and to assess the threshold independently.

Artefact rejection facilities.   Apart from off-line methods of artefact rejection, it is advantageous to exclude high random voltages by an on-line method so that the total number of single responses contributing to the averaged waveform is kept fairly constant. The simple method discussed in Chapter Two may be used.

Permanent recording of averaged responses.   The averaged responses can be permanently traced on to paper or photographed, then several people can be asked to decide on the level of the threshold. It helps considerably, when judging whether a response is positive or not, to be able to compare the amplitudes and latencies of the waveform with those obtained at a slightly higher intensity.

Testing procedures

Adult subjects and older children may be tested lying on a couch or sitting with the neck supported. Young children must be tested under sedation as any movements will produce myogenic electrical artefacts. Mendel, Adkinson and Harker (1974) tested infants during natural sleep but evidence (Kupperman and Mendel, 1974) suggests that sedatives may be used and that light sleep is best for the recording of responses (REM or stages I or II).

The electrodes are placed on the vertex of the scalp and on the contralateral mastoid process with the earthing electrode situated usually, on the forehead. The stimuli are delivered from an earphone. The determination of theshold at several frequencies often requires a 2 to 3 hour test session. Several trials are necessary using the same stimulus at near to threshold intensity levels so that a judgement on whether responses are present 50 per cent of the time can be reached. To many clinicians, this long test period is unattractive.

Results of recent clinical work

Practically all the work on the middle latency responses has been directed towards its use as a means of estimating the auditory threshold.

Goldstein and Rodman (1967) published the first favourable report showing a close correlation between the auditory threshold and the threshold of the responses. It was hoped, therefore, that middle latency responses could be used to predict the hearing levels of young children whilst they slept peacefully. The reports concerning children are, however, contradictory. Mendel *et al.* (1974) evaluated the responses in 18 infants and obtained identifiable responses within 15 to 30 dB HL in most cases. Lowell (1965) and Davis and Hirsh (1973), both found the middle latency responses to be difficult to evaluate in young children and preferred the slow cortical responses (CERA). It is likely, furthermore, that the middle latency responses undergo a maturation of the waveform in the first few months of life and, until further work has been done, it is difficult to interpret the responses of the very young. At present, it cannot be said that the middle latency responses have left the laboratory stage and, with the advent of ECochG and BER, it seems unlikely that they will ever have widespread clinical use.

As a means of neuro-otological diagnosis, the middle latency responses could have real value. Robinson and Rudge (1977) found latency abnormalities but not amplitude abnormalities in patients with multiple sclerosis.

Final remarks

The work on the middle latency responses has almost exclusively been performed at the University of Wisconsin by Goldstein and his collaborators and more recently in Iowa by Mendel and his colleages. Despite the fact that there is still some doubt as to which components are entirely neurogenic and which contain some myogenic components, it does appear that these responses can provide a means of ERA. The advantage of the responses is that they are not altered much by light sleep, but this advantage is also shared by ECochG and BER. The disadvantages are that careful analysis of the results is necessary before a threshold can be estimated, and the reliability of the responses is poor compared with ECochG and BER (it is possible for a child to be diagnosed as having a hearing loss when he is merely a 'poor responder'). The length of the test period and the frequent difficulties in interpretation of the results diminish the clinical value of using middle latency responses for screening children.

Appendix 1. Glossary

The following definitions have been selected from the British Standard Glossary of Acoustical Terms, BS 661. The definitions are reproduced by permission of the British Standards Institution, 2, Park Street, London, W.1, from whom copies are obtainable. For full information, the complete standard should be consulted.

Acoustics
a) **The science of sound.**
b) **Of a room or auditorium. Those factors that determine its character with respect to the quality of the received sound.**

Amplitude
Of a simple sinusoidal quantity. The peak value.

Audiogram
A chart or table relating hearing level for pure tones to frequency.

Audiometer
An instrument for measuring hearing acuity.

Bel
A scale unit used in the comparison of the magnitudes of powers. The number of bels, expressing the relative magnitudes of two powers, is the logarithm to the base 10 of the ratio of the powers.

Binaural hearing
1. Normal perception of sounds and/or of their directions of arrival with both ears.
2. By extension, the perception of sound when the two ears are connected to separate electro-acoustic transmission channels.

Cycle
Of a periodic quantity. The sequence of changes which takes place during the period of a recurring variable quantity.

Decibel
One-tenth of a bel. Abbreviation dB.
  Note 1: Two powers P_1, and P_2 are said to be separated by an interval of n·bels (or 10n decibels) when $n = \log_{10}(P_1/P_2)$.

Note 2: When the conditions are such that the ratios of sound particle velocities and ratios of sound pressures (or analogous quantities such as electric currents or voltages) are the square roots of the corresponding power ratios the number of decibels by which the corresponding powers differ is expressed by the following formulae:

$$n = 20 \log_{10}(u_1/u_2)dB$$
$$n = 20 \log_{10}(P_1/P_2)dB$$

where u_1/u_2 and P_1/P_2 are the given sound particle velocity and sound pressure ratios respectively.

By extension a single magnitude of any of these quantities may be expressed in decibels relative to a stated reference magnitude (it being understood that no impedance change is concerned). Thus for example the sensitivity of a microphone may be expressed either as:

        x volts per Pa

or as   y dB relative to 1 volt per Pa

where $y = 20 \log_{10} x$.

Earphone
Telephone receiver
An electro-acoustic transducer operating from an electrical system to an acoustical system and designed to be applied to the ear.

Frequency
Of a period quantity. The rate of repetition of the cycles. The reciprocal of the period. The unit is the hertz. Symbol f.

Note: Frequency may be expressed in hertz (Hz), kilohertz (kHz) or megahertz (MHz).

Harmonic
Of a non-sinusoidal periodic quantity. A sinusoidal component of the periodic quantity having a frequncy which is an integral multiple of the fundamental frequency.

Note: In physics and electrical engineering the nth harmonic implies a frequency equal to n times the fundamental frequency: in music the nth harmonic usually implies a frequency equal to (n+1) times the fundamental frequency.

Headphone
Head receiver
An earphone attached to a head band by which it is held to the ear.

Hearing level
Hearing threshold level
A measured threshold of hearing expressed in decibels relative to a specified standard of normal hearing.

Hearing loss
The increase of individuals' hearing level above the specified standard of normal hearing when this can be ascribed to a specific cause such as advancing age, conductive deafness, perceptive defects or noise exposure.

Impedance

Acoustic impedance
Of a specified configuration or medium. The complex ratio of the sound pressure to the volume velocity through a chosen surface. Symbol Za.

Characteristic impedance
Of a medium in which sound waves are propagated. The specific acoustic impedance at a point in a progressive plane wave propagated in the medium.
Note: In the case of a non-dissipative medium the characteristic impedance is equal to pc.

Specific acoustic impedance
Unit area impedance
At a point in a sound field. The complex ratio of the sound pressure to the particle velocity. Symbol Zs.

Insert earphone
Insert receiver
An earphone of small dimensions associated with a fitting for insertion into the auditory meatus.

Level
Of a quantity related to power. The ratio, expressed in decibels, of the magnitude of the quantity to a specified reference magnitude.

Level recorder
An instrument for registering, usually logarithmically, the variation with time of the magnitude of an electrical signal.
Note: The input is frequently derived from a microphone.

Loudness
An observer's auditory impression of the strength of a sound.

Loudness level
The loudness level of a sound is measured by the sound pressure level of a standard pure tone of specified frequency which is assessed by normal observers as being equally loud.

Masking
a. The process by which the threshold of hearing of one sound is raised due to the presence of another.
b. The increase, expressed in decibels, of the threshold of hearing of the masked sound due to the presence of the masking sound.

Microphone
An electro-acoustic transducer operating from an acoustical system to an electrical system.

Monaural hearing
The perception of sound by stimulation of a single ear.

Noise
Sound which is undesired by the recipient. Undesired electrical disturbances in a transmission channel or device may also be termed 'noise', in which case the qualification 'electrical' should be included unless it is self-evident.

Normal threshold of hearing
The modal value of the thresholds of hearing of a large number of otologically normal observers between 18 and 25 years of age.

Peak value
Of a varying quantity in a specific time interval. The maximum numerical value attained whether positive or negative.

Perceived noise level
The perceived noise level of a sound is measured by the sound pressure level of a reference sound which is assessed by normal observers as being equally noisy. The reference sound consists of a band of random noise between one-third and one octave wide centred on 1000 Hz.

Pitch
That attribute of auditory sensation in terms of which sound may be ordered on a scale related primarily to frequency.

Presbyacusis
Hearing loss mainly for high tones due to advancing age.

Pure tone
A sound in which the sound pressure varies sinusoidally with time. The waveform may be represented by a siniot.

Pure tone audiometer
An instrument for measuring hearing acuity to pure tones by determination of hearing level.

Recruitment
An aspect of certain forms of perceptive deafness, whereby the growth of loudness of a sound with its sound pressure level is greater than it is for normal subjects.

Root mean square value
(r m s value) Effective value — Of a varying quantity. The square root of the mean value of the squares of the instantaneous values of the quantity. In the case of a periodic variation the mean is taken over one period.

Sensation level
Of a specified sound. The sound pressure level when the reference sound pressure corresponds to the threshold of hearing for the sound.

Sound
a. Mechanical disturbance, propagated in an elastic medium, of such character as to be capable of exciting the sensation of hearing.

By extension, the term 'sound' is sometimes applied to any disturbance, irrespective of frequency, which may be propagated as a wave motion in an elastic medium.

Disturbances of frequency too high to be capable of exciting the sensation of hearing are described as ultrasonic. Hypersonics is the name given to ultrasonic disturbances in a medium, whose wavelength is comparable with the intermolecular spacing.

Disturbances of frequency too low to be capable of exciting the sensation of hearing are described as infrasonic.

b. The sensation of hearing excited by mechanical disturbance.

Sound intensity
In a specified direction. The sound energy flux through unit area, normal to that direction; symbol I.

Note: It is customary to define the area parallel to the wave front, in which case $I = P^2/\rho c$ for a plane or spherical free progressive wave, where p is the density. (P = sound pressure: c = volocity of sound.)

Sound level
A weighted value of the sound pressure level as determined by a sound level meter.

Sound level meter
An instrument designed to measure a frequency-weighted value of the sound pressure level. It consists of a microphone, amplifier and indicating instrument having a declared performance in respect of directivity, frequency response, rectification characteristic, and ballistic response.

Sound pressure
At a point in a sound field. The alternating component of the pressure at the point. The unit is the pascal (Pa).

Note: The term sound pressure may be qualified by the terms 'instantaneous', 'peak', 'maximum', r m s , etc. The r m s sound pressure is frequently understood by the unqualified term sound pressure; symbol P.

Sound pressure level
The sound pressure level of a sound, in decibels, is equal to 20 times the logarithm to the base 10 of the ratio of the r.m.s. sound pressure to the reference sound pressure. In case of doubt, the reference sound pressure should be stated.

In the absence of any statement to the contrary, the reference sound pressure in air is taken to be 2×10^{-5} Pa (equals 2×10^{-4} dyn/cm^2) and in water 0.1 Pa (equals 1 dyn/cm^2).

Sound wave
A disturbance whereby energy is transmitted in a medium by virtue of the inertial, elastic and other dynamical properties of the medium. Usually the passage of a wave involves only temporary departure of the state of the medium from its equilibrium state.

Speech audiometer
An instrument for the measurement of hearing by means of live or recorded speech signals.

Threshold of hearing
Threshold of audibility — Of a continuous sound. The maximum r m s value of the sound pressure which excites the sensation of hearing.

Tinnitus
A subjective sense of 'noises in the head' or 'ringing in the ears'.

Tone
a) A sound giving a definite pitch sensation.
b) Sometimes, also, the physical stimulus giving rise to the sensation.

Transducer
A device designed to receive oscillatory energy from one system and to supply related oscillatory energy to another.
   Note: In acoustics one system is usually electrical, the other usually acoustical or mechanical.

Waveform
The shape of the graph representing the successive values of a varying quantity, usually plotted in a rectangular co-ordinate system.

Wavelength
Of a sinusoidal plane progressive wave. The perpendicular distance between two wavefronts in which the phases differ by one complete period. Symbol λ
   Note: The wavelength is equal to the phase velocity divided by the frequency.

PART 2. ELECTRONIC DEFINITIONS

Amplifier
Device which produces a higher signal output power, output voltage, or output current than that applied to its input.
Analogue
In an analogue system or an analogue computer the signal varies in a similar (or analogous) way to the physical quantity being measured. (Contrast with digital.)

Attenuator
Device which reduces the amplitude of a signal.

Calibration
The placing of appropriate marks on a scale, such as the frequency scale of a radio receiver.

Circuit
Group of wires or electronic components around which an electric current can flow.

Comparator
High gain integrated circuit amplifier, designed for comparing two input voltages. Normally provides an output voltage which is either 'high' or 'low' according to which of the input voltages has the greater value.

Computer

Equipment which can carry out mathematical operations on the information fed into it. It may use either analogue or digital techniques.

Cross talk

In a stereo system any signal in one channel may appear in the other channel at a greatly reduced amplitude; this is known as cross talk. For example, if one sees in a circuit specification 'cross talk – 70dB', this means that any signal in one channel may produce the same signal in the other channel at a level of 70dB lower than in the original channel.

Cycles per second

Cycles per second (or hertz, Hz) is a measure of frequency. For example, the mains frequency in the U.K. is 50Hz. This means that the mains voltage changes its polarity and returns to its original polarity fifty times per second.

Differential amplifier

Two signals can be fed to a different amplifier, the output depending on the difference between the two signals. Thus any stray signals, such as hum, which are present at both inputs will not appear at the output to any significant extent.

Digital

A digital system is one in which any signal is represented as a series of pulses. Digital systems are used in computing and in radio and television systems between the studio and transmitters. The signal is unaffected by disortion unless a whole pulse is lost or a noise pulse is accepted as a signal pulse.

Electrode

A point at which an electric current enters or leaves a device or a cell.

Feedback

A signal taken from the output of an amplifier may be fed back and added to the input signal. If it re-inforces the input, the feedback is positive and oscillation may occur. If the feedback subtracts from the input signal, it is negative; the gain is reduced, but so is the distortion.

Filter

A circuit which allows signals of a certain frequency to pass easily through it, but attenuates signals of certain other frequencies. A high pass filter transmits signals above a certain frequency with little attenuation, but attenuates lower frequencies; a low pass filter has the opposite effect. A bandpass filter passes a certain band of frequencies.

Frequency modulation (fm)

A method of carrying information by a radio frequency wave in which the frequency of the carrier is changed in sympathy with the aduio frequency modulating waveform.

Gain

The amplification provided by a circuit. One may refer to voltage gain or power gain.

Gate
A circuit which allows certain signals to pass through it to other circuits, whilst it rejects other signals.

Hertz (Hz)
The unit of frequency. The mains power supply alternates 50 times per second and is therefore said to have a frequency of 50Hz.

Micro (μ)
Prefix placed in front of a unit meaning one millionth.

Milli (m)
A prefix which can be placed in front of unit to reduce its value by one thousant times.

Ohm
The unit of resistance, named after the German physicist G.S. Ohm. An object has a resistance of 1 ohm when a potential difference of 1V placed across it causes a current of.1S to flow through it.

Oscilloscope
An instrument which permits the waveform of a voltage to be displayed as a trace on the screen of a cathode ray tube. Small signals can be amplified before being displayed.

Peak-to-peak
The peak-to-peak voltage of an alternating current waveform is the voltage difference between the uppermost part of the waveform and the lowest negative part of it.

Polarity
Direction in which a voltage is applied across a device.

Potential
Potential (more correctly potential difference, p.d.) is equivalent to the voltage across a device or between two points in a circuit.

Preamaplifier
An amplifier placed before the main amplifier. The signal levels in a preamplifier are often very low and it is vital to employ a very low noise preamplifier.

Rise time
Time taken by a pulse to rise from 10% of its maximum height to 90% of its maximum height.

Sensitivity
The greater the sensitivity of a meter or of a receiver, the smaller the signal it can respond to.

Signal
A signal carries information. In the electronics field, a signal is normally a constant or an alternating voltage or current or one or more pulses.

Waveform
The way voltage or current at a point in a circuit changes with time. A waveform can be displayed on an oscilloscope screen.

Wavelength
The distance between two peaks or two other identical points of a wave. For all waves, velocity = wavelength × frequency. The normal symbol for wavelength is λ (lambda).

White noise
Consists of a mixture of equal parts of all audible frequencies, like white light consists of all colours. It sounds like a hiss, most of the energy being in the high frequency regions which occupy almost all of the bandwidth.

PART 3. SPECIFIC DEFINITIONS

An averaged response
A response which consists of the average of many individual responses.

Dead ear
An ear without any auditory or vestibular function. (Slang otological term)

Epoch
A specific period of time. (In ERA, this usually refers to the period during which the subject's biological signals are being fed into the averaging system.)

Electric (or evoked) response audiometry
The method of audiometry involving the analysis of the biological evoked electrical events occurring after sound stimulation.

Off-line analysis
Analysis of the data from a recorded source after the actual test period.

On-line analysis
Analysis of the data during the actual test period.

Primary cortical response
The first wave of electrical activity occurring in a specific area of the cortex after stimulation.

Secondary cortical response
Waves of electrical activity occurring after the primary cortical response from a wide area of the cortex.

Sub-threshold stimulation
Stimulation of insufficient intensity to be perceived.

Supra-threshold stimulation
Stimulation of sufficient intensity to be perceived.

Temporal auditory summation
The process by which the response to or the perception of a sound increases as the duration of the sound is extended.

Appendix 2 Further Notes Concerning Stimulus Intensity Calibration

The calibration of the intensity of the stimuli used for ERA is of great importance. There are many problems in calibrating transient acoustic stimuli and it was felt worthwhile to add some further remarks in addition to those already made in Chapter 2. These remarks are merely of an introductory nature.

Four different methods of calibrating the stimulus intensity are commonly found in ERA literature. These are based on the following measurements:

Physical measures
1. Sound pressure level
2. Peak equivalent level

Biological measures
3. Hearing level
4. Sensation level

PHYSICAL MEASUREMENTS

1. Sound pressure level

The sound pressure level (SPL) of a sound or noise is conveniently measured in decibels (dB). The number of decibels is equal to 20 times the logarithm to the base 10 of the ratio of the root mean square (rms) sound pressure to the reference sound pressure. In the case of the weighting scales, the reference level at OdB at 1000 hertz (Hz) is a sound pressure level of 0.0002 dynes/cm². (One dyne is the force which will accelerate a mass of one gramme at a rate of one centimetre per second per second. Recently some workers have prefered the SI unit, pascals (Pa), which are ten times larger than dynes/cm²).

The threshold of hearing for a sound of given character is the minimal value which excites the sensation of hearing. The SPL weighting scales have been designed to reflect normal hearing levels. At the upper and lower frequency ranges of the auditory spectrum higher sound pressures are needed to effect hearing. Obviously the hearing threshold varies according to the age and otological condition of the subject. Normal values are based on the modal data from groups of supposedly normal-hearing subjects. There are several methods of selecting such groups and so there are three different SPL weighting curves in current use. ERA workers most commonly seem to·employ the dB A scale.

The disadvantage of the SPL weighting scales lies with the difficulties in measuring accurately the SPL of a transient. Even if a SPL meter is used with a very fast response, it is likely that the reading will only reveal a certain proportion of the sound energy actually within the transient. The accuracy with which the SPL meter reflects the true sound energy depends on the quality (and expense) of the meter's construction.

Table 1 compares the weighing values of different SPL scales.

Table 1. Responses, in dB., are expressed relative to the response at 1000Hz.
(0.0002 dynes/cm² or 20μ Pa)

Frequency Hz	Curve A dB	Curve B dB	Curve C dB	Curve D dB
31.5	−39.4	−17.1	−3.0	−16.5
50	−30.2	−11.6	−1.3	−12.5
80	−22.5	−7.4	−0.5	−9.0
100	−19.1	−5.6	−0.3	−7.5
125	−16.1	−4.2	−0.2	−6.0
250	−8.6	−1.3	0	−2.0
500	−3.2	−0.3	0	0
1000	0	0	0	0
2000	1.2	−0.1	−0.2	8.0
4000	1.0	−0.7	−0.8	11.0
8000	−1.1	−2.9	−3.0	6.0
16000	−6.6	−8.4	−8.5	−4.0

Table reproduced in part from International Electrotechnical Commission (1965) Publication 179, 1st Ed., 'Precision sound level meters.' Geneva, IEC.

These measurements are made using an acoustic coupler which presents a specified acoustic impedance to the earphone which is not directly related to the mean acoustic impedance of the average human ear.

2. Peak equivalent sound pressure level

One method of overcoming the problem of measuring accurately the SPL of a transient acoustic stimulus is by comparing the maximum peak to peak amplitude of the transient to the peak to peak amplitude of a pure tone stimulus of a known SPL. This method is accurate in a physical sense but bears little relation to the concept of normal hearing lying at 0dB level. The more transient the stimulus, the greater the SPL required to reach the psychoacoustic threshold and the wider the discrepancy between dB pe SPL and the biological calibration of clinical audiometers.

It is not possible to provide a table comparing the values of the dB pe SPL scale to those of the biological scale (dB ISO) as there are too many variable factors. Usually the psycho-acoustic threshold lies at a figure between 30-45dB on the pe SPL scale.

BIOLOGICAL MEASUREMENTS

The audiometers used clinically are calibrated according to a biological specification. The reference zero (0dB) is determined by the normal threshold. The normal threshold refers to the threshold of hearing at the specified frequency using a specified type of earphone. The normal value is a modal value determined by testing an adequately large number of otologically normal subjects within the age limits of 18-25 years of age. An otologically normal subject is a person in a normal state of health who is free from all signs or symtoms of ear disease and from wax in the ear canal and has no history of undue noise exposure.

It is not practical to calibrate every audiometer by testing large numbers of normal subjects. Each audiometer is calibrated using an arteficial coupler or, better, an arteficial ear which has been designed to measure the exact amount of sound pressure emitted by the specified earphone. The standards set for this calibration method have been developed over the past thirty years.

The first reference zero was established in the United States of America and the values were based on the determinations of the hearing threshold in 'normal' ears reached in the United States National Health Survey in 1937. The results were expressed in terms of a Western Electric Type 705A earphone using the American Standards Association's 9A acoustic coupler. The details are explained in the 1951 specification for Audiometers for General Diagnostic Purposes (ASA Z24.3–1951). Fifteen years later, the British established their own reference zero based on laboratory studies conducted in England in 1952. These studies were performed using more modern equipment, in better acoustic conditions and using better psycho-acoustic techniques than the earlier American study. As a consequence, the British Standard (BS 2497, 1954), which applied to an arteficial ear conforming to BS 2042 (1953) and ST and C type 4026A earphones, was approximately 10dB more sensitive than the American standard.

It was clearly undesirable that there should be two different standards and as a consequence the International Standards Organisation met and determined a standard which was agreeable to both the British and to Americans. The results of 15 different studies were considered (almost half these studies were performed in the United States) and the agreement between all the studies was excellent. After several years of discussion and calculation these data were combined to form the International Standard Reference Zero for the uniform calibration of all pure tone audiometers. The standard was approved unanimously by the Council of the ISO in 1963 and the recommendation was published in 1964 (ISO R389). Later an addendum was produced (ISO r389: 1970) which allowed the ISO reference zero to be determined using several different artifial ears or acoustic couplers and various types of earphone. There were still some difficulties as the earphones used commercially were not the ones used for standardisation but further work has been accomplished and there are now several tables available which cover a wide range of earphones.

3. Hearing level

The ISO recommendations (R389) apply only to pure tone stimuli of a duration of at least 0.5 seconds and not to transient stimuli. It is not possible to calibrate the brief stimuli used for the short latency ERA responses using an arteficial ear according to ISO standards. Nevertheless most clinicians are now familiar with this scale and it is an advantage to use a calibration scale which bears resemblance.

It is possible to calibrate transients according to a hearing level (HL) zero standard. The common practice is to use a group of normal hearing subjects aged 18–25 years and to determine the mean hearing threshold for this group for each of the stimuli to be used for ERA purposes. There are some obvious problems since at suprathreshold levels, loudness will differ when the subjects have certain pathological conditions. Nevertheless this biological method of calibrating transient stimulus intensity does escape from many of the pitfalls encountered on using a physical method of calibration.

4. Sensation level

The subject's own psycho-acoustic threshold may be used as the reference zero. This method of calibration is acceptable when normative ERA studies are undertaken but is not very useful for clinical work.

The publications mentioned are available upon request from—

The British Standards Institute, 2 Park Street, London W1;
The American Standard Association, 10, East 40th Street, New York 16.

Appendix 3 Operating instructions and some typical switch positions for users of the Medelec/Amplaid Mk III ERA equipment

The apparatus used by the author to obtain the various recordings shown in the original figures in this book was the Medelec/Amplaid Mk III ERA equipment. This equipment is commercially available. As many clinics possess the same equipment, it was thought that it might be helpful to list the actual switch positions commonly used by the author. Anyone beginning work with this apparatus should be able to reproduce easily the recordings illustrated by simply using the same switch positions. Admittedly, it is not absolutely necessary to follow exactly all the switch positions listed as there are many different switch positions which also give satisfactory results. Once experience has been gained, it is likely that the tester will wish to introduce many modifications of his own.

The account which follows gives switch positions in an abbreviated form but it should prove comprehensible to readers who use the Medelec/Amplaid equipment. The figures in circles, viz: ③ relate to the diagram of the apparatus (fig 3.1).

GENERAL NOTES

First switch the apparatus **ON**!

Selecting the oscilloscope sweep period

Choose an oscilloscope sweep period which is appropriate to the response to be averaged. Recommended periods for ECochG, BER and CERA are listed later in this appendix.

The sweep velocity for each division is selected by using the switch bank ⑥ immediately below the oscilloscope display. If there are 8 divisions on the screen multiply the figure chosen by 8 to calculate the total sweep period for display.

Using the timing scale

If the equipment incorporates **two AA6 Mk II or Mk III** amplifiers, it is possible to use one to give a continuous time scale display on the oscilloscope screen whilst the other is used to amplify the patient's signal. Then each averaged response which is photographed will be accompanied by a time scale which makes subsequent analysis of the data much easier (see Fig. 8.1).

Switch positions
  AA6 Mk II amplifiers ⑩ & ⑪ : determine which amplifier is connected with

195

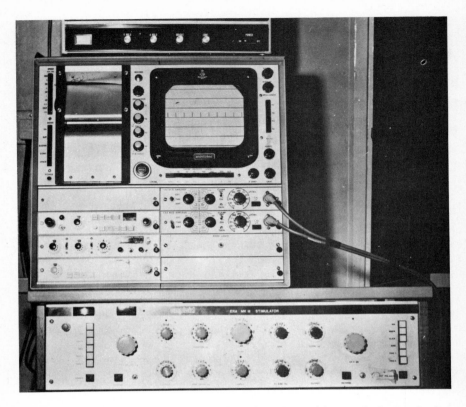

channel one and place the switch on the far left to the position marked **t** (or **time**). Next adjust the position of the timing scale to the lower edge of the oscilloscope display by turning**Y4** ④. (Channel 2 is used to monitor the patient's signals).

AA6 Mk III amplifiers (not illustrated): this appendix describes the Mk II amplifier settings in all the ensuing notes but those workers using the more recently introduced Mk III amplifiers should have no difficulty in adapting the instructions.

Averaging the responses

Attach the necessary electrodes to the subject and insert the free ends into the pre-amplifier associated with channel 2. Switch the pre-amplifier **ON.** Select channel 2 on the averager expander ⑨.

Before commencing it is wise to check the quality of the signal arriving from the patient by using **Y2** ④ on the oscilloscope display. It is also possible to listen to this signal by operating the controls to the right of the oscilloscope display ⑤.

The averaging can be performed **automatically** to a pre-set number of individual responses (epochs) or, **manually,** when averaging is stopped by the operator whenever he wishes.

Switch positions

Automatic: select the required number of epochs to be averaged on the **DAV6** unit ⑧ using the centrally-placed control.

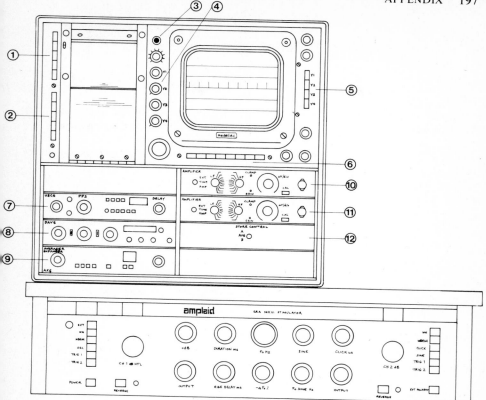

Press momentarily the start/stop switch (between the erase and reject buttons) into the **down** position.

After the pre-set number of epochs, the machine automatically stops. The number of epochs is displayed on the indicator immediately above the start/stop switch.

The averaged response on the oscilloscope display **Y4** ④ can be enlarged or decreased by altering the number of averages (divisions) made by the DAV6 unit. Turn the gain switch (immediately to the left of the erase button) to the required position. Write the number of epochs and the gain setting, together with the details of the stimulus used, onto the photographed trace for future reference.

Manual: sometimes it is helpful to watch the averaged response building on the oscilloscope display. For example, place the gain control switch to 64 for EcochG or BER and then operate the start stop switch into the upward position. When an averaged response of the required amplitude has been obtained, return the start/stop switch to the central position. Do not forget it is easier for later calculations to finish the recording on exponent number, eg 512 or 1024, and remember to write the details down.

Photographing the data

The traces displayed on the oscilloscope can be photographed onto Kodak linagraph direct print paper (type 1895). This paper develops itself on exposure to light. If the paper is exposed too long to light, it over-develops or fogs. The paper will also fog immediately if subjected to the light from a photographer's flash bulb.

A small black container which clips to the front of the photographic unit may be used to prevent any exposure of the paper to light so that it can be chemically developed and fixed at a later date.

Switch positions
Ignore all the switches in the upper switch bank ①.

Press **SPACE** ② lightly several times until a length of unexposed paper extrudes and write on this the details of the patient (age, hospital number, name, diagnosis etc.). The author usually writes a complete abstract of the patient's clinical notes as experience has taught him that this may be the last occasion that he may be able to find the notes!

For economic use, press **SS** (single shot) **IN** only. The photographs will be tightly spaced. If **SPACE** is also pressed **IN**, there will be a gap between each photograph which can be used for writing notes.

The photograph is taken by either pressing a switch ③ on the machine or by using a foot switch.

Erasing the averaged response
After each averaged response has been recorded and photographed, erase it from the memory of the DAV6 and from oscilloscope display by pressing **both** the erase and reject buttons ⑧.

Calibrating the averaged response amplitude
Do not forget to calibrate the traces obtained by recording and photographing the calibration pulse using the same amplifier gain as used during the recording session.

Switch positions
Switch **OFF** the pre-amplifier.
Press **IN** the calibration button on the **AA6 MkII** amplifier ⑪
Average the calibration pulse using the **DAV6** ⑧
Photograph the calibration pulse on **Y2** ④ and the averaged calibration pulse on **Y4** ④ of the oscilloscope display.

NOTES FOR SPECIFIC RESPONSES

Electrocochleography

Electrodes
Active (transtympanic) to **RED** pre-amp input.
Reference (earlobe) to **BLACK** pre-amp input.
Earth (forehead-inion) to **GREEN** pre-amp input.

Switch positions
Pre-amp check switch is **ON**
(check patient's signal on **Y2**)

Sweep velocity ⑥: choose a 10 ms sweep period by pressing **IN** the switches to give a **1.25ms/div** sweep volocity.

AA6 Mk II amplifier ⑪ : use the amplifier connected with channel 2. Set **LF** to 50ms or 3.2Hz. Set **HF** to 3.2K (kHz). Switch **CLAMP OFF**. Turn the switch on the far left of the module to position marked **AMP** or **AA6**. Leave the calibration switch **OUT**. The usual gain setting is **20μV/div**, but it is better to turn the gain switch as far clockwise as possible without the rejection indicator above the start/stop switch ⑧flashing on too frequently.

Either **US62** ⑦: This unit controls the number of stimuli presented to the patient each second. For ECochG purposes, **10pps** (pulses per second is usually selected, but **20pps** may be selected to shorten the period of testing when threshold work is undertaken. The desynch switch may be used if there is any danger of contamination from mains interference. Press **GATED IN**. Press **GROUP SHIFT IN**, unless the loudspeaker is being used, as this gives a useful pre-stimulus delay of about 2.2ms. Press **TRIG 1 IN**. There is no need to operate any other switches in this module except if you wish to use the latency measuring facility.

Or **AS62** (not shown in Fig. A3.1): This unit is less expensive than the US62 module and is incorporated into the apparatus in some centres. The instructions are nearly similar to those for the US62 unit. Select **10pps** or **20pps** as wished. Random **IN** if necessary. **TRIG 1** is pressed **IN. PROGRAMME** switch is pressed **IN**. Do not operate any of the other switches on this unit.

DAV6 ⑧: set **DELAY** dial to **0′** and make sure that the accompanying slide switch to the right is in the **CENTRAL** position. Select an **ANALYSIS TIME** of **10ms** and check that its accompanying slide switch is in the **CENTRAL** position. Usually 256 epochs have to be averaged and a gain multiplication factor of 4 is needed but these figures vary a great deal.

Store control switch ⑫ : place this switch in the **CENTRAL** positions which is not marked **A** or **B**.

Averager expander ⑨: select **CHANNEL 2 IN** and press **ALT IN**.

The dial on the far right of the module selects the data to be displayed on the oscilloscope screen (**Y4**). Normally, during ECochG, the settings reveal the following data:

A+B shows the action potential and the summating potential complex (AP/SP) with the cochlear microphonic suppressed.

A–B shows the cochlear microphonic (CM) with the AP/SP complex suppressed.

A shows the CM and AP/SP obtained to the stimuli which began in one particular phase or polarity.

B shows the CM and AP/SP complex to the stimuli in the opposite polarity to those of B.

ALT shows the A and B traces alternately.

Audiometer (Amplaid Mk III model): use the right-hand section.

Press **TRIG 1 IN**

Select either **CLICK** or **SINE** and press **IN** as appropriate. If **CLICK** is chosen, use a **100μs duration**. If **SINE** is chosen, usually **4** sine waves is appropriate for ECochG work but this number does depend on the frequency selected.

Select the **FREQUENCY** if sine waves were chosen.

Press **EXT POLARITY IN**

Turn the intensity dial to the required **INTENSITY** which is then shown on the display.

Use **PHN** (the special earphone) whenever possible, otherwise use the loudspeaker.

Averaging the responses may now commence according to the instructions given in the general notes of this appendix. The following traces should appear on the oscilloscope display:

Y1 should show a timing scale.

Y4 should show the data selected by the averager expander.

Y2 shows the unaveraged (raw) signal from the patient. This trace generally should be removed from the display before each photograph is taken.

Y3 shows the response to half the total number of stimuli delivered and is identical with **Y4** when the averager expander selects A. It is not generally included on the display during ECochG.

Removing the SP component from the AP/SP waveform

All switches are operated in the same manner as described for ECochG with the following exceptions:

Audiometer: the best subtraction results are obtained on using a stimulus of either 2kHz, 8 sine waves or 4kHz, 16 sine waves. Select an intensity which provides a clear AP/SP waveform.

Next follow this sequence:

Store control switch: select **B**

US62 or *AS62*: select **100pps** but check the actual timing with a stopwatch as it rarely is exactly 100 per second. **Random** switch must be **OUT**.

Sweep velocity: alter the sweep velocity to *100μs/div* as this provides an 8ms display period.

Averager expander: select **B**.

Then average the responses **MANUALLY** until a number of approximately 256 or 512 has been reached. Now begin the second stage of the proceedure:

Store control switch: this is altered to **A**.

US62 or AS62: change to **5pps**

Averager expander: alter to **A**.

Averaging now recommences, **WITHOUT ERASING**, until a figure is reached which is exactly double that averaged during the first stage. After averaging is completed, the oscilloscope display **Y4** will provide the following traces:

Averager expander

A shows the full amplitude AP with SP

B shows mainly SP as the AP is attenuated due to the fast stimulus presentation rate.

A–B shows the AP less that part of it still apparent on **B** but the SP or similar DC components are completely suppressed.

Brainstem electrical responses

Electrodes

Active (mastoid) to **RED** pre-amp input

Reference (vertex or forehead, in midline immediately below hairline) to **BLACK** pre-amp input

Earth (inion or chin) to **GREEN** pre-amp input

Switch positions

Pre-amp: check switch is **ON**

(check patient's signal on Y2)

Sweep velocity ⑥: choose a 16 ms sweep period by pressing **IN** the switches to give a *200μs/div* sweep velocity

AA6 Mk II amplifier ⑪ : use the amplifier connected with channel 2. Set **LF** to

250 Hz (this filter setting is not a standard fixture on the unit and has to be added). Set **HF** to **3.2K** (kHz). Switch the **CLAMP OFF**. Leave the calibration switch **OUT**. Turn the switch on the far left of the module to the position marked **AMP** or **AA6**. The gain control setting should be **5μV/div** but occasionally the signal is too large, rejection occurs as shown by the red light flashing on the DAV6 ⑧ module, and the gain setting has to be turned to **10μV/div**.

Either *US62* ⑦: Use **20pps** for threshold purposes and use **10pps** for neuro-otological purposes as the slower rate shows all the various BER peaks more clearly. Use the random switch as wished. Press **GATED IN**. Press **GROUP SHIFT IN**, as this provides a pre-stimulus analysis period of about 2.5ms. Press **TRIG 1 IN**. The author usually uses the latency marker to show the 6ms analysis mark on the oscilloscope display as this is the position where the NV of the BER waveform first becomes apparent.

Or *AS62* (not shown in Fig. A3.1): Basically the instructions are similar to those for using the **US62** with the following exceptions: there is no **GROUP SHIFT. PROGRAMME** is pressed **IN** in place of **GATED**.

DAV6 ⑧: set **DELAY** dial to **0** and make sure that the accompanying slide switch to the right is in the **CENTRAL** position. Select an **ANALYSIS TIME** of **20ms** and check that the accompanying slide switch is in the **CENTRAL** position. Usually 2048 epochs must be averaged manually with a gain multiplication factor of 32 but these figures vary.

Store control switch ⑫ : during the first 1024 epochs this is placed in position **A** and during the subsequent epochs (total epochs 2048) the **B** position is selected. The switch position is changed when the figure 1024 is indicated on the **DAV6** display without stopping the averaging. This manouevre helps check the reliability of the BER.

Averager expander ⑨: select **CHANNEL 2 IN**. It does not matter whether **ALT** is **IN** or **OUT**. The dial on the far right of the module selects the data shown on the oscilloscope screen (**Y4**). The settings should reveal the following data:

A The BER waveform to the first 1024 stimuli
B The BER waveform to the second 1024 stimuli
ALT Displays the reliability as **A** and **B** are shown alternately. Ideally, the two traces should superimpose exactly.
A+B shows the BER waveform to all 2048 stimuli
A–B should ideally be almost a straight line if the response reliability is really good.

Audiometer (Amplaid Mk III model): use the right-hand section.
Press **TRIG 1 IN**. Press **SINE IN**.
Leave **EXT POLARITY OUT**; the green light should be off.
Turn the stimulus polarity control switch situated on the top surface of the audiometer at the rear to unipolarity Ω.
Select the desired **FREQUENCY** between 1kHz and 8kHz.
Choose **2** or **4** sine waves.
Turn the intensity dial to the required stimulus intensity as indicated by the display above this control.
The best BER waveform is obtained using the special earphone (**PHN**). Sometimes masking of the non-test ear is necessary. Unless the test is conducted in an anechoic chamber, the loudspeaker may cause acoustical reverberations which confuse the BER recordings.

Averaging the response: Averaging is performed manually according to the instructions in the general notes of this appendix. The following traces should appear on the display:

Y1 should show the timing scale

Y4 should show the BER waveform as selected by the averager expander.

Y2 shows the patient's signal and it is not generally included onto the photograph.

Y3 shows the BER waveform to alternate stimulus presentations and provides yet another method of checking the response reliability.

Cortical ERA

Electrodes
Active (vertex) to **RED** pre-amp input.
Reference (on either mastoid) to **BLACK** pre-amp input.
Earth (forehead-inion) to **GREEN** pre-amp input.

Switch positions
Pre-amp: check switch is **ON**.
(check patient's signal on Y2)

Sweep velocity ⑥: choose a **70ms/div** sweep velocity which gives a 560ms sweep period on the display.

AA6 Mk II amplifier ⑪ : use the amplifier connected with channel 2. Set **LF** to **100ms** or **1.6Hz**. Set **HF** to **10ms** or **16Hz**. Switch the **CLAMP OFF**. Turn the switch on the far left of the module to position marked **AMP** or **AA6**. Leave the calibration switch **OUT**. The usual gain setting is **50µV/div**, but it is best to turn the gain switch as far clockwisw as possible without the rejection indicator above the start/stop switch ⑧ flashing on too frequently.

Either *US62* ⑦: This unit controls the number of stimuli presented to the patient each second. For CERA purposes, 1pps (pulse per second) is usually selected. The **RANDOM** switch should be pressed **IN**. Press **GATED IN**. Press **GROUP SHIFT IN** as this provides a useful pre-analysis delay of about 125ms. Press **TRIG 1 IN**. There is no need to operate any other switches on the module except if one wishes to use the latency measuring facility.

Or *AS62* (not shown in Fig. A3.1): The operation of this unit is very similar to that of the **US62** unit, except: there is no **GROUP SHIFT** facility but a delay of 100ms can be arranged by using the DAV6 unit ⑧. **PROGRAMME** is pressed **IN** instead of **GATED**.

DAV6 ⑧: if the **US62** unit is being used, there is not need to use the delay facilities on this module; set **DELAY** dial to **0** and make sure that the accompanying slide switch to the right is in the **CENTRAL** position. If the **AS62** unit is being used, choose a delay of 100ms by turning the **DELAY** dial to **10** and moving the accompanying switch on the right of the dial to **x10**. Select an **ANALYSIS TIME** of 600ms, by turning the dial to **60** and the accompanying slide switch to the right to **x10**. Usually 32 or 64 epochs have to be averaged and a gain multiplication factor of 8 is needed but these figures vary on testing different subjects.

Store control switch ⑫ : it is useful to retain a response in **A** whilst averaging the next response in **B**. The first response may act as a useful template for judging the presence or absence of the second response. Unfortunately, there is no facility for erasing **A** or **B** independently so once both **A** and **B** have been filled, the entire display has to be erased. Alternatively, it is often helpful to use the same technique as described for **BER** and store the first half of the epochs recorded in **A** and the second half of the epochs in **B**. A and **B** may then be compared for reliability

Averager expander ⑨: select **CHANNEL 2 IN**. It does not matter whether **ALT** is **IN** or **OUT**. The dial on the far right selects the data shown on the oscilloscope screen (**Y4**). It depends entirely on how the store control switch was used as to what data is shown on turning the dial to the various positions. For example, if **A** was used to store the first half of an averaged response to 64 stimuli and then the store control switch was turned quickly to **B** so the remainder of the response was stored in **B**, the settings should reveal the following data:

A The CERA to the first 32 stimuli
B The CERA to the following 32 stimuli
A+B The CERA to all 64 stimuli.

ALT shows traces A and B and these should ideally superimpose exactly but rarely does this occur in practice.

A–B should be a straight line if the response reliability is absolute.

Audiometer (Amplaid Mk III model): use the left-hand section.

Press **OSC IN**

Press **TRIG 1 IN**

Select **BURST**. Set the appropriate dials to provide a burst of **30ms DURATION** and **20ms RISE/DECAY**.

Select the **FREQUENCY** by turning the large centrally-placed dial. **1kHz** is usually a very suitable frequency for commencing the test. Choose the stimulus intensity (**dB**) by using the large dial on the left and watching the display immediately above this control.

Use the TDH 39 earphones and place the **RED** earphone over the subject's right ear. The settings on the audiometer, **L** (left) and **R** (right) may be selected for testing the appropriate ear. Small children must be tested using the loudspeaker. Masking of the non-test ear is often necessary.

Averaging the responses may now commence according to the instructions in the general notes of this appendix. The following traces should appear on the oscilloscope display.

Y1 should show the timing scale. The lower dots occur at 10ms intervals and the upper dots at 100ms interval.

Y2 shows the unaveraged (raw) signal from the patient.

Y3 shows the responses averaged in the **A** store.

Y4 should show the CERA, according to the selection of data chosen using the averager expander.

In conclusion

It is hoped that these notes will prove comprehensible to workers using the Medelec/Amplaid Mk III equipment. By following the instructions exactly, it should be possible to operate the equipment satisfactorily and to obtain ECochG, BER or CERA responses. It may be useful to ask a colleague to read the instructions for a particular response and to set each switch position as it is read. After some practice, the operation of the equipment becomes easy to understand and, it is expected, that the tester will wish to introduce many of his own modifications.

Bibliography

Abé, M. (1954) Electrical responses of the human brain. *Tohôku Journal of Experimental Medicine,* **60,** 47-58.

Ades, W. H. & Brookhart, J. M. (1950) The central auditory pathway. *Journal of Neurophysiology,* **13,** 189-205.

Ades, H. W., Engström, H. & Hawkins, J. E. Jr. (1962) Structure of inner ear sensory epithelial cells in relation to their functions. BUMED project MR 005-13-2005, Pensacola Fla. Naval School of Aviation Medicine. Report No. 1.

Adrian, E. D. (1926) The impulses produced by sensory nerve endings. *Journal of Physiology,* **61,** 49-72.

Adrian, E. D. & Matthews, B. H. C. (1934) The Berger rhythm: potential changes from the occipital lobes in man. *Brain,* **57,** 355-385.

Andreev, A. M., Arapova, A. A. & Gerusuni, S. V. (1939) On the electrical potentials of the human cochlea. *Journal of Physiology (USSR),* **26,** 205-212.

Antinoro, F. & Skinner, P. (1968) The effects of frequency on the auditory evoked response. *Journal of Auditory Research,* **8,** 119-123.

Antinoro, F., Skinner, P. & Jones, J. (1969) Relation between sound intensity and amplitude of the auditory evoked response at different stimulus frequencies. *Journal of the Acoustical Society of America,* **46,** 1433-1436.

Appleby, S. V. (1964) The slow vertex maximal sound evoked response in infants. *Acta Oto-laryngologica,* Supplementum **206,** 146-152.

Antonelli, A. R. (1976) Electrophysiological measures of auditory perception. *Revue de Laryngologie,* **97,** Supplementum, 613-621.

Aran, J. M., Charlet de Sauvage, R. & Pelerin, J. (1971) Comparison des seuls électrocochléographiques et de l'audiogramme. Etude statistique. *Revue de Laryngologie,* **92,** 477-491.

Aran, J. M., Darouzet, J. & Erre, J. P. (1975) Observations of quick evoked compound eighth nerve responses before, during and over seven months after kanamycin treatment in guinea pigs. *Acta Oto-laryngologica,* **79,** 24-32.

Arlinger, S. D. (1976a) N1 latencies of the slow auditory evoked potential. *Audiology,* **15,** 370-375.

Arlinger, S. D. (1976b) Auditory responses to frequency ramps—a psychoacoustic and electrophysiological study. *Linköping University Medical Dissertations,* **No. 40.** Linköping.

Ashcroft, P. B., Humphries, K. N. & Douek, E. E. (1975) New developments in the use of the crossed acoustic response as a screening test in children. Paper read at The Second British Conference on Audiology, Southampton.

Bamford, J. M. (1977) A note on the use of the terms 'subjective' and 'objective' in audiology. *British Journal of Audiology,* **11,** 19-21.

Bancaud, J., Bloch, V. & Paillard, J. (1953) Contribution EEG a l'étude des potentiels évoques chez l'homme au niveau du vertex. *Revue de Neurologie,* **89,** 382-399.

Barnes, W. T., Magoun, H. W. & Ranson, S. W. (1943) Ascending auditory pathway in the brainstem of monkey. *Journal of Comparative Neurology,* **79,** 129-152.

Barnet, A. B. & Goodwin, R. S. (1965) Averaged evoked electroencephalographic responses to clicks in the newborn. *Electroencephalography and Clinical Neurophysiology,* **18,** 441-450.

Barr, B. (1955) Pure tone audiometry for pre-school children. *Acta Oto-laryngologica,* Supplementum **121.**

Bauhin, C. (1605) Theatrum anatomicum. Francofurti at Moenum. Cited by Wever, E. G. in *Theory of Hearing.* New York: John Wiley.

Beagley, H. A. (1965) Acoustic trauma in the guinea pig ll. Electron microscopy including the morphology of cell functions in the organ of Corti. *Acta Oto-laryngologica,* **60,** 479-495.

Beagley, H. A. (1971) Present day scope and limitations of evoked response audiometry. *Revue de Laryngologie.* Supplementum 753-763.

Beagley, H. A. (1972) Progress in objective audiometry. *Journal of Laryngology and Otology*, **86**, 225-235.

Beagley, H. A. (1973) Electrophysiological methods in the diagnosis and management of deafness. *Minerva Otorhinolaryngologica*, **23**, 173-181

Beagley, H. A. (1974) Personal communication.

Beagley, H. A., Fateen, A. M. & Gordon, A. G. (1972) Clinical experience of evoked response and subjective auditory thresholds. *Sound*, **6**, 8-13.

Beagley, H. A. & Gibson, W. P. R. (1974) ERA in the diagnosis and treatment of hearing-impaired children. Paper read at VIII Curso Monografico y I Curso-Symposium Internacional sobre Nuevas Technicas de Exploracion Auditiva, Seville.

Beagley, H. A. & Gibson, W. P. R. (1976) Lesions mimicking acoustic neuroma using transtympanic electrocochleography. In *Disorders of Auditory Function II*, edited by S. D. G. Stephens, pp. 119-125. London: Academic Press.

Beagley, H. A., Hutton, J. N. T. & Hayes, R. A. (1974) Clinical electrocochleography: a review of 106 cases. *Journal of Laryngology and Otology*, **88**, 993-1000.

Beagley, H. A. & Kellogg, S. E. (1968) A comparison of evoked response and subjective auditory thresholds. *International Audiology*. **7**, 420-421.

Beagley, H. A. & Knight, J. J. (1967) Changes in auditory evoked response with intensity. *Journal of Laryngology and Otology*, **81**, 861-873.

Beagley, H. A., Legouix, J.P., Teas, D.C. & Remond, M.C. (1977). Changes in ECochG in acoustic neuroma, some experimental findings. *Clinical Otolaryngology*. **2**, 213-219.

Beiter, R. C. & Hogan, D. D. (1973) Effects of variations in stimulus rise-decay time upon the early components of the auditory evoked response. *Electroencephalography and Clinical Neurophysiology*, **34**, 203-206.

Békésy, G. von (1944) Über die mechanische frequenzanalyze der schnecke vershiedener tiere. *Akustica Zietschrift*, **9**, 2-11.

Békésy, G. von (1947) The variation of phase along the basilar membrane with sinusoidal vibrations. *Journal of the Acoustical Society of America*, **19**, 452-462.

Békésy, G. von (1950) D-C potentials and energy balance of the cochlear partition. *Journal of the Acoustical Society of America*, **22**, 576-582.

Békésy, G. von (1951) The coarse pattern of the electrical resistance in the cochlea of the guinea pig (electroanatomy of the cochlea). *Journal of the Acoustical Society of America*, **23**, 18-28.

Békésy, G. von (1952) D-C resting potentials inside the cochlea partition. *Journal of the Acoustical Society of America*. **24**, 72-76.

Békésy, G. von & Rosenblith, W. A. (1951) The mechanical properties of the ear. In *Handbook of Experimental Psychology*, edited by S. S. Stevens, Chapter 27. New York: John Wiley.

Berger, H. (1929) Über das elektroenkephalogramm des menschen. *Archives für Psychiatrie und Nervenkrankheiten*, **87**, 527-570.

Berger, H. (1930) Über das elektroenkephalogramm des menschen: zweite mitteilung. *Journal für Psychologie und Neurologie*, **40**, 160-179.

Berlin, C. I., Cullen, J. K., Ellis, M. S., Lousteau, R. J. & Yarborough, W. M. (1974) Clinical application of recording VIII nerve action potentials from the tympanic membrane. *Trans-American Academy for Ophthalmology and Otolaryngology*, **78**, ORL 401-410.

Best, G. La Var & Tabor, J. R. (1968) Cortical audiometry as an otological proceedure. *Trans-American Academy for Ophthalmology and Otolaryngology*, **72**, 142-152.

Bevan, J. (1971) The human auditory evoked response and contingent negative variation in hyperbaric air. *Electroencephalography and Clinical Neurophysiology*. **30**, 198-204.

Bickford, R. G. (1966) Human microreflexes revealed by computer analysis. *Neurology*. **16**, 302.

Bickford, R. G., Galbraith, R. F. & Jacobson, J. L. (1963a) The nature of average evoked potentials recorded from the human scalp. *Electroencephalography and Clinical Neurophysiology*. **15**, 720.

Bickford, R. G., Jacobson, J. L. & Galbraith, R. F. (1963b) A new audiomotor system in man. *Electroencephalography and Clinical Neurophysiology*. **15**, 922.

Bickford, R. G., Jacobson, J. L. & Cody, D. T. R. (1964) Nature of average evoked potentials to sound and other stimuli in man. *Annals of the New York Academy of Science*, **112**, 204-223.

Bickford, R. G., Sem-Jacobsen, C. W., White, P. & Daly, P. (1952) Symposium: photo-metrazol activation of the electroencephalogram; some observations on the mechanism of photic and photo-metrazol activation. *Electroencephalography and Clinical Neurophysiology*, **4**, 275-282.

Bochenek, Z. & Bochenek, W. (1975) Early (12–16ms) responses evoked by tones and clicks. *Revue de Laryngologie*, **96**, 115-120.

Blegvad, B. (1976) Binaural summation of surface recorded electrocochleographic responses. *Scandinavian Audiology*, **4**, 233-238.

Bordley, J. E. (1956) An evaluation of the psychogalvanic skin-resistance technique in audiometry. *Laryngoscope*, **66**, 1162.

Bordley, J. E. & Hardy, W. G. (1949) A study in objective audiometry with the use of a psychogalvanometric response. *Annals of Otology, Rhinology and Laryngology*, **58**, 751-760.

Bordley, J. E., Hardy, W. G. & Richter, C. P. (1948) Audiometry with use of galvanic skin-resistance response; preliminary report. *Bulletin of the John Hopkins Hospital*, **82**, 569.

Borsanyi, S. J. & Blanchard, C. L. (1964) Auditory evoked brain responses in man. *Archives of Otolaryngology*, **80**, 149-154.

Bostem, F., Rousseau, J. C., Degossely, M. & Dongier, M. (1967) Psychopathological correlates of the non-specific portion of visual and auditory evoked potentials and the associated contingent negative variation. *Electroencephalography and Clinical Neurophysiology*. Supplementum **26**, 131-138.

Brackmann, D. (1975) Personal communication.

Brugge, J. F., Anderson, D. J., Hind, J. E. & Rose, J. E. (1969) Time structure of discharges in single auditory nerve fibres of the squirrel monkey in response to complex periodic sound. *Journal of Neurophysiology*, **32**, 386-401.

Brummett, R. E., Meikle, M. M. & Vernon, J. A. (1971) Ototoxicity of tobramycin in guinea pigs. *Archives of Otolaryngology*, **94**, 59-63.

Brummett, R. E., Himes, D., Saine, B. & Vernon, J. A. (1972) A comparative study of the ototoxicity of tobramycin and gentamicin. *Archives of Otolaryngology*, **96**, 505-512.

Bryant, G. (1976) The effect of sedatives upon the waveform of the brainstem auditory potentials. Unpublished BSc thesis. University of London.

Buchwald, J. S. & Huang, C. H. (1975) Far-field acoustic response: origins in the cat. *Science*, **189**, 382-384.

Burian, K. (1975) The influence of sedation on the evoked potential their identification in routine ERA. *Revue de Laryngologie*, **96**, 176-177.

Burian, K. & Gestring, G. F. (1971) Discrepancies between subjective and objective acoustic thresholds. *Archiv für Klinische und Experimentelle Ohren —Nasen —und Kehlkopfheilkunde*, **198**, 73-82.

Burian, K., Gestring, G. F., Gloning, K. & Haider, M. (1972) Objective examination of verbal discrimination and comprehension in aphasia using contingent negative variation. *Audiology*, **11**, 310-316.

Burian, K., Gestring, G. F. & Haider, M. (1969) Objective speech audiometry. *International Audiology*, **8**, 387-390.

Burian, K., Gestring, G. F. & Hruby, S. (1970) Evoked response audiometry under sedation. *Electroencephalography and Clinical Neurophysiology*, **28**, 215.

Butler, R. A., Konishi, T. & Fernández, C. (1960) Temperature coefficents of cochlear potentials. *American Journal of Physiology*, **199**, 688-692.

Cajal, S. Ramon y (1909) In *Histologie du systeme nerveux de l'homme et des vertebres*. Paris: A. Maloine.

Campbell, A. W. (1905) In *Histological studies on the localisation of cerebral function*. Cambridge-University Press.

Cant, B. R. & Bickford, R. G. (1967) The effect of motivation on the contingent negative variation (CNV). *Electroencephalography and Clinical Neurophysiology*, **23**, 594.

Caspers, H. (1961) Changes of cortical DC potentials in the sleep-wakefulness cycle. In *The Nature of Sleep*, edited by G. E. W. Wolstenholme and C. M. O'Conner. pp. 237-253. Boston: Littlebrown.

Caton, R. (1875) The electric currents of the brain. Abstract. *British Medical Journal*, **ii**, 278.

Cazals, Y. & Stephens, S. D. G. (1975) The loudness function for click stimuli. *Journal of Auditory Research*, **15**, 95-105.

Celesia, G. G., Broughton, R. J., Rasmussen, T. & Branch, C. (1968) Auditory evoked responses from the exposed human cortex. *Electroencephalography and Clinical Neurophysiology*, **24**, 458-466.

Chang, H-T. (1950) The repetitive discharges of cortico-thalamic reverberating circuit. *Journal of Neurophysiology*, **13**, 235-257.

Charlet de Sauvage, R. & Aran, J. M. (1973) L'Electrocochléogramme normal. *Revue de Laryngologie*, **94**, 93-107.

Chatrian, G. E., Petersen, M. C. and Lazarte, J. A. (1960) Responses to clicks from the human brain:

some depth electrographic observations. *Electroencephalography and Clinical Neurophysiology*, **12**, 479-489.

Chiorini, J. R. (1969) Slow potential changes from cat cortex during classical aversive conditioning. Doctoral dissertation: University of Iowa.

Chow, K. L. (1951) Numerical estimates of the auditory central nervous system of the rhesus monkey. *Journal of Comparative Neurology*, **95**, 159-175.

Clark, W. A. Jr. (1958) Average response computer (ARC-1). *Quarterly Progress Report No.49 Research laboratory of electronics. Massachusetts Institute of Technology. Cambridge, Massachusetts: MIT press.*

Clark, J. A. Jr., Goldstein M. H. Jr., Brown, R. M., Molnar, C. E., O'Brien, D. F. & Zieman, H. E. (1961) The average response computer (ARC): a digital device for computing averages and amplitudes and time histograms of electrophysiological responses. *Transactions of I. R. E.*, **8**, 46-51.

Clarke, G. P. (1976) Personal communication.

Claus, H., Handrock, M. & Arentsschild, O. (1975) Comparison between conventional audiometry and ERA for deaf children in a serial test. *Revue de Laryngology*, **96**, 133-137.

Clayton, L. G. & Rose, D. E. (1970) Auditorily evoked cortical responses in man and recruiting ears. *Journal of Auditory Research*, **10**, 79-81.

Coats, A. C. (1964a) Physiological observation of auditory masking. I Effect of masking duration. *Journal of Neurophysiology*, **27**, 988-1000.

Coats, A. C. (1964b) Physiological observation of auditory masking II Effect of masking intensity. *Journal of Neurophysiology*, **27**, 1001-1010.

Coats, A. C. (1967) Physiological masking in the peripheral auditory system III Effect of varying click intensity. *Journal of Neurophysiology*, **30**, 931-948.

Coats, A. C. (1971) Depression of click action potential by attenuation, cooling and masking, *Acta Oto-laryngologica*, Supplementum **284**.

Coats, A. C. & Dickey, J. R. (1970) Nonsurgical recording of human auditory nerve potentials and cochlear microphonics. *Annals of Otology, Rhinology and Laryngology*, **79**, 844-852.

Cody, D. T. R. & Bickford, R. G. (1969) Averaged evoked myogenic responses in normal man. *Laryngoscope*, **79**, 400-416.

Cody, D. T. R., Griffing, T. & Taylor, W. F. (1968) Assessment of the newer tests of auditory function. *Annals of Otology, Rhinology and Laryngology*, **77**, 686-705.

Cody, D. T. R., Jacobson, J. L., Walker, J. C. & Bickford, R. G. (1964) Averaged evoked myogenic and cortical potentials to sound in man. *Annals of Otology, Rhinology and Laryngology*, **73**, 763-777.

Cody, D. T. R. & Klass, D. W. (1968) Cortical audiometry: potential pitfalls in testing. *Archives of Otolaryngology*, **88**, 396-406.

Cody, D. T. R. & Townsend, G. L. (1973) Some physiologic aspects of the averaged vertex response in humans. *Audiology*, **12**, 1-13.

Cohen, J. (1969) Very slow brain potentials relating to expectancy: the CNV. In *Average Evoked Potentials—methods, results and evaluations,* edited by E. Donchin, & D. B. Lindsley, 143-198. NASA symposium 191. Washington DC: US government printing office.

Cohen, J. & Walter, W. G. (1966) The interaction of responses in the brain to semantic stimuli. *Psychophysiology*, **2**, 187-196.

Cohen, M. H., Rapin, I., Lyttle, M. & Schimmel, H. (1971) Auditory evoked response (AER): Consistency of detection in young sleeping children. *Archives of Otolaryngology*, **94**, 214-219.

Cotugno, D. (1761) *De aquae ductibus auris humanae internae* Neapoli: ex. typ. Simonianca.

Crowley, D. E., Davis, H. & Beagley, H. A. (1975) Survey of the clinical use of electrocochleography. *Annals of Otology, Rhinology and Laryngology*, **84**, 1-11.

Cullen, J. K. Jr., Ellis, M. S., Berlin, C. I. & Lousteau, R. J. (1972) Human acoustic nerve action potential recordings from the tympanic membrane without anaesthesia. *Acta Oto-laryngologica*, **74**, 15-22.

Daigneault, E. A. (1974) Source of the P1 component of the cochlea round window potential. *Acta Oto-laryngologica*, **77**, 405-411.

Dallos, P. (1972) Cochlear potentials. A status report. *Audiology*, **11**, 29-41.

Dallos, P. (1973) Cochlear potentials and cochlear mechanics. In *Basic Mechanisms of Hearing,* edited by A. R. Moller, and P. Boston, pp 335-376. New York: Academic press.

Dallos, P. (1975) Cochlear potentials. In *The Nervous System,* edited by D. B. Tower. Volume 3 *Human Communication and its Disorders.* pp. 69-80. New York: Raven Press.

Dallos, P. (1976) Personal communication.

Dallos, P. & Cheatham, M. A. (1976) Compound action potential (AP) tuning curves. *Journal of the Acoustical Society of America*, **59**, 591-597.

Dallos, P., Schoeny, Z. G. & Cheatham, M. A. (1972) Cochlear summating potentials: descriptive aspects. *Acta Oto-laryngologica*. Supplementum **302**.

David, S. & Sohmer, H. (1972) Experiments on cats to determine the nature of the auditory evoked response in man. *Israel Journal of Medical Sciences*, **8**, 571.

Davis, H. (1951) Psychophysiology of hearing and deafness. In *Handbook of Experimental Psychology*, edited by S. S. Stevens, New York: John Wiley.

Davis, H. (1960) Mechanisms of excitation of auditory nerve impulses. In *Neural Mechanisms of the Auditory and Vestibular Systems*, edited by G. L. Rasmussen, and W. F. Windle, Ch. 2. Springfield: Thomas.

Davis, H. (1961) Some principles of sensory receptor action. *Physiological Revue*, **41**, 391-416.

Davis, H. (1964) Enhancement of evoked cortical potentials in humans related to a task requiring a decision. *Science*, **145**, 182-183.

Davis, H. (1965a) Sonomotor reflexes: myogenic evoked potentials. In *The Young Deaf Child: Identification and Management*, edited by H. Davis, *Acta Oto-laryngologica*, supplementum 206, 122-124.

Davis, H. (1965b) Slow cortical responses evoked by acoustic stimuli. *Acta Oto-laryngologica*, **59**, 179-185.

Davis, H. (1968) Mechanisms of the inner ear. *Annals of Otology, Rhinology and Laryngology*, **77**, 644-656.

Davis, H. (1971) Round table conference on terminology. *Archiv für Klinische und Experimentelle Ohren—Nasen—und Kehlkopfheilkunde*, **198**, 167-176.

Davis, H. (1972) Classes of auditory evoked responses. Paper read at The Eleventh International Congress of Audiology, Budapest.

Davis, H. (1973) Sedation of young children for electric response audiometry (ERA). *Audiology*, **12**, 55-57.

Davis, H. (1975) Personal communication.

Davis, H. (1976a) Principles of electric response audiometry. *Annals of Otology, Rhinology and Laryngology*, **85**, supplementum 28.

Davis, H. (1976b) Brainstem and other responses in electric response audiometry. *Annals of Otology, Rhinology and Laryngology*, **85**, 3-14.

Davis, H., Davis, P. A., Loomis, A. L., Harvey, E. N. & Hobart, G. (1939) Electrical reactions of the human brain to auditory stimulation during sleep. *Journal of Neurophysiology*, **2**, 500-514.

Davis, H., Deatherage, B., Eldredge D. H. & Smith, C. A. (1958a) Summating potentials of the cochlea. *American Journal of Physiology*, **195**, 251-261.

Davis, H., Eldredge, D. H. & Gannon, R. P. (1958b) Some effects of electrical polarisation of the organ of Corti. *Physiologist (London)*, **1**, 15.

Davis, H., Engebretson, M., Lowell, E. L., Mast, T., Satterfield, J. & Yoshie, N. (1963) Evoked responses to clicks recorded from the human scalp. *Annals of the New York Academy of Sciences*, **112**, 224-225.

Davis, H., Fernández, C. & McAuliffe, D. R. (1950) The excitatory process in cochlea. *Proceedings of the National Academy of Sciences. U.S.A.*, **36**, 580-587.

Davis, H. & Hirsch, S. K. (1973) Clinical trial of fast responses in ERA. Paper read at The Third Symposium of the International ERA Study Group, Bordeaux.

Davis, H. & Hirsch, S. K. (1975) Brain-stem responses to 500Hz signals. Paper read at The Fourth Symposium of the International ERA Study Group, London.

Davis, H., & Hirsch, S. K. (1976) The audiometric utility of brain-stem responses to low-frequency sounds. *Audiology*, **15**, 181-195.

Davis, H. & Hirsch, S. K. (1977) ERA of young children at 500Hz. Paper read at the Fifth Symposium of the International ERA study group, Jérusalem.

Davis, H., Hirsch, S. K., Shelnutt, J. & Bowers, C. (1967) Further validation of evoked response audiometry (ERA). *Journal of Speech and Hearing Research*, **10**, 717-732.

Davis, H., Mast, T., Yoshie, N. & Zerlin, S. (1966) The slow response of the human cortex to auditory stimuli: recovery process. *Electroencephalography and Clinical Neurophysiology*, **21**, 105-113.

Davis, H. & Onishi, S. (1969) Maturation of auditory evoked potentials. *International Audiology*, **8**, 24-33.

Davis, H., Osterhammel, P. A., Wier, C. C. & Gjerdingen, D. B. (1972) Slow vertex potentials: interaction among auditory, tactile, electric and visual stimuli. *Electroencephalography and Clinical Neurophysiology*, **33**, 537-545.

Davis, H. & Yoshie, N. (1963) Human evoked cortical responses to auditory stimuli. *The Physiologist*, **6**, 164.

Davis, H. & Zerlin, S. (1966) Acoustic relations of the human vertex potential. *Journal of the Acoustical Society of America*, **39**, 109-116.

Davis, P. A. (1939) Effects of acoustic stimuli on the waking human brain. *Journal of Neurophysiology*, **2**, 494-499.

Dawson, G. D. (1947) Cerebral responses to electrical stimulation of peripheral nerve in man. *Journal of Neurology, Neurosurgery and Psychiatry*, **10**, 134-140.

Dawson, G. D. (1950) Cerebral responses to nerve stimulation in man. *British Medical Bulletin*, **6**, 326-329.

Dawson, G. D. (1951) A summation technique for detecting small signals in a large irregular background. *Journal of Physiology*, **115**, 2P-3P.

Dawson, G. D. (1954) A summation technique for the detection of small evoked potentials. *Electroencephalography and Clinical Neurophysiology*, **6**, 65-84.

De Boer, E. (1969) Reverse correlation II. Initiation of nerve impulses in the inner ear. *Proceedings: Koninklijke Nederlandse Akademie van Wetenschappen; Senesc, Biological and Medical Sciences.* **72**, 129-151.

Derbyshire, A. J. & McDermott, M. (1958) Further contributions to the E.E.G. method of evaluating auditory function. *Laryngoscope*, **68**, 558-570.

Desmedt, J. E. (1962) Auditory evoked potentials from cochlea to cortex as influenced by activation of the efferent olivo-cochlear bundle. *Journal of the Acoustical Society of America*, **34**, 1478-1496.

Dix, M. R., Hallpike, C. S. & Hood, J. D. (1948) Observations upon the loudness recruitment phenomenon, with especial reference to the differential diagnosis of disorders of the internal ear and VIIIth nerve. *Journal of Laryngology and Otology*, **62**, 671-686.

Doerfler, L. G. (1948) Neurophysiological clues to auditory acuity. *Journal of Speech and Hearing Disorders*, **13**, 227-232.

Donald, M. W. & Goff, W. R. (1971) Attention-related increases in cortical responsivity dissociated from CNV. *Science*, **172**, 1163-1166.

Donchin, E., Tueting, P., Ritter, W., Kutas, M. & Heffley, E. (1975) On the independence of the CNV and the P300 components of the human averaged evoked potential. *Electroencephalography and Clinical Neurophysiology*, **38**, 449-461.

Douek, E. E., Ashcroft, P. B. & Humphries, K. N. (1976) The clinical value of the post-auricular myogenic (crossed acoustic) responses in neuro-otology. In *Disorders of Auditory Function II*, edited by S. D. G. Stephens, pp. 139-143. London: Academic Press.

Douek, E. E. & Clarke, G. P. (1976) A single average crossed acoustic response. *Journal of Laryngology and Otology*, **90**, 1027-1032.

Douek, E. E., Gibson, W. P. R. & Humphries, K. N. (1973) The crossed acoustic response. *Journal of Laryngology and Otology*, **87**, 711-726.

Douek, E. E., Gibson, W. P. R. & Humphries, K. N. (9174) The crossed acoustic response and objective tests of hearing. *Developmental Medicine and Child-Neurology*, **16**, 32-39.

Douek, E. E., Gibson, W. P. R. & Humphries, K. N. (1975) The crossed acoustic response. *Revue de Laryngologie*, **96**, 121-125.

Downman, C. B. B., Woolsey, C. N. & Lende, R. A. (1960) Auditory areas I, II and EP: cochlear representation, afferent paths and interconnections. *Bulletin of the John Hopkins Hospital*, **106**, 127-142.

Du Verney, J. G. (1683) *Traite de l'organe de l'ouie.* Paris: E. Michallet.

Economopoulou, H., Krogh, H. J. & Fosvig, L. (1970) EEG-computer audiometry (ERA) in a group of pre-school and school-age children. *Acta Otolaryngologica*, supplementum **263**, 248-250.

Eggermont, J. J. (1976) Tuning curves for normal and pathological human cochleas. Paper read at The Thirteenth International Congress of Audiology, Florence.

Eggermont, J. J. & Don, M. (1977) Results of high-pass masking; brainstem responses vs auditory nerve APs. Paper read at V symposium of International ERA study group. Jerusalem.

Eggermont, J. J., & Odenthal, D. W. (1974a) Frequency selective masking in electrocochleography. *Revue de Laryngologie*, **95**, 489-495.

Eggermont, J. J. & Odenthal, D. W. (1974b) Methods in electrocochleography. *Acta Otolaryngologica*, supplementum **316**, 17-24.

Eggermont, J. J. & Spoor, A. (1973a) Cochlear adaptation in guinea pigs (a quantitative description). *Audiology*, **12**, 193-220.

Eggermont, J. J. & Spoor, A. (1973b) Masking of action potentials in the guinea pig cochlea, its relation to adaptation. *Audiology*, 12, 221-241.

Elberling, C. (1973) Transitions in cochlear action potentials recorded from the ear canal in man. *Scandanavian Audiology*, 2, 151-159.

Elberling, C. (1974) Action potentials along the cochlear partition recorded from the ear canal in man, *Scandanavian Audiology*, 3, 13-19.

Elberling, C. (1976a) Action potentials recorded from the promontory and the surface, compared with recordings from the ear canal in man. *Scandanavian Audiology*, 5, 69-79.

Elberling, C. (1976b) High frequency evoked action potentials recorded from the ear canal in man. *Scandanavian Audiology*, 5, 157-164.

Elberling, C. (1976c) Deconvolution of action potentials recorded from the ear canal in man. In *Disorders of Auditory Function II*, edited by S. D. G. Stephens, pp. 109-117. London: Academic Press.

Elberling, C. & Salomon, G. (1971) Electrical potentials from the inner ear in man in response to transient sounds generated in a closed acoustic system. *Revue de Laryngologie*, supplementum, 691-707.

Engel, R. & Young, N. (1969) Calibrated pure tone audiograms in neonates based on evoked electroencephalographic responses. *Neuropaedatrics*, 1, 149-160.

Engström, H. (1958) On the double innervation of the sensory epithelia of the inner ear. *Acta Otolaryngologica*, 49, 109-118.

Engström, H. (1960) The cotilymph, the third lymph of the inner ear. *Acta Morphologica. Neerl-Scand*, 3, 195-208

Engström, H., Ades, H. W. & Hawkins, J. E. (1965) Cellular pattern, nerve structures and fluid spaces. In *Contributions to Sensory Physiology, Volume 1*, edited by W. D. Neff, pp. 1-37. New York: Academic Press.

Engström, H. & Fernàndez, C. (1961) Discussion to Smith, C. A. *Trans-American Otological Society*, 49, 58.

Erulkar, S. D. (1959) The responses of single units of the inferior colliculus of the cat to acoustic stimulation. *Proceedings of the Royal Society, series B (Biological Sciences)*, 150, 336-355.

Evans, E. F. (1972) The frequency response and other properties of single fibres in the guinea-pig cochlear nerve. *Journal of Physiology*, 226, 263-287.

Evans, E. F. (1975a) Normal and abnormal functioning of the cochlear nerve. In *Sound Reception in Mammals*, edited by R. J., Bench, A. Pye, and J. E. Pye, pp. 133-165. London: Academic Press.

Evans, E. F. (1975b) The sharpening of cochlear frequency selectivity in the normal and abnormal cochlea. *Audiology*, 14, 419-442.

Evans, E. F., Rosenberg, J. & Wilson, J. P. (1970) The effective bandwidth of cochlear nerve fibres. *Journal of Physiology*, 207, 62P-63P.

Evans, E. F. & Wilson, J. P. (1973) Frequency selectivity of the cochlea. In *Basic Mechanisms of Hearing*, edited by A. R. Moller and P. Boston, pp. 519-551. New York: Academic Press.

Feré, C. (1888) Note sur des modifications de la résistance electrique sous l'influences des excitations sensorielles et des emotions. *Comptes Rendus des Séances de la Société de Biologie (Paris)*, 5, 217.

Ferriss, G. S., Davis, G. D., Dorsen, M. McF. & Hackett, E. R. (1967) Changes in latency and form of the photically induced averaged evoked response in human infants *Electroencephalography and Clinical Neurophysiology*, 22, 305-312.

Freeman, J. (1965) Monitoring psychomotor response to stress by evoked auditory responses. USAF School of Aerospace Medicine, Airospace Medical Division (AFSC), Report SAM-TR-65-42. Texas: Brooks Airforce Base.

Friedman, D., Simson, R., Ritter, W. & Rapin, I. (1975) Cortical evoked potentials elicited by real speech words and human sounds. *Electroencephalography and Clinical Neurophysiology*, 38, 13-19.

Fromm, B., Nylen, C. O. & Zotterman, Y. (1935) Studies in the mechanism of Wever-Bray effect. *Acta Oto-laryngologica*, 22, 477-486.

Furukawa, T. & Ishii, Y. (1967) Neurophysiological studies on hearing in goldfish. *Journal of Neurophysiology*, 30, 1378-1403.

Gabor, D. (1947) Acoustical quanta and the theory of hearing. *Nature*, 159, 591-594.

Galambos, R. (1956a) Some recent experiments on the neurophysiology of hearing. *Annals of Otology, Rhinology and Laryngology*, 65, 1055-1059.

Galambos, R. (1956b) Suppression of auditory nerve activity by stimulation of efferent fibres to the cochlea. *Journal of Neurophysiology,* 19, 424-437.

Galambos, R. & Davis, H. (1948) Action potentials from single auditory-nerve fibres? *Science,* 108, 513.

Galambos, R., Schwartzkopff, J. & Rupert, H. (1959) Microelectrode study of superior olivary nuclei. *American Journal of Physiology,* 197, 527-536.

Galley, N., Klinke, R., Oertel, W., Pause, M. & Storch, W-H. (1973) The effects of intracochlearly administered acetylcholine-blocking agents on the efferent synapses of the cochlea. *Brain Research,* 64, 55-63.

Garner, W. R. (1947) Auditory thresholds of short tones as a function of repetition rates. *Journal of the Acoustical Society of America,* 19, 600-608.

Gastaut, Y. (1953) Les points negatives evoquées sur le vertex. Leur signification psycho-physiologique et pathologique. *Revue de Neurologie,* 89, 382-399.

Gavilan, C. & Sanjuan, J. (1964) Microphonic potential picked up from the human tympanic membrane. *Annals of Otology, Rhinology and Laryngology,* 73, 101-109.

Geisler, C. D. (1960) Average responses to clicks in man recorded by scalp electrodes. Technical report, no. 380. Research laboratory of electronics, Massachusetts Institute of Technology. Cambridge, Massachusetts: MIT press.

Geisler, C. D. (1964) In discussion. *Annals of the New York Academy of Science,* 112, 218-219.

Geisler, C. D., Frishkopf, L. S. & Rosenblith, W. A. (1958) Extracranial responses to acoustic clicks in man. *Science,* 128, 1210-1211.

Gibson, W. P. R. (1974) *Investigations of the post-auricular myogenic responses.* Unpublished MD thesis: University of London.

Gibson, W. P. R., & Beagley, H. A. (1976a) Electrocochleography in the diagnosis of acoustic neuroma. *Journal of Laryngology and Otology,* 90, 127-140.

Gibson, W. P. R. & Beagley, H. A. (1976b) Transtympanic electrocochleography in the investigation of retro-cochlear disorder. *Revue de Laryngologie,* 97, supplementum, 507-517.

Gibson, W. P. R. & Beagley, H. A. (1977) Differences between the broad component contributions to the ECochG responses obtained from patients with either Ménière's disorder or acoustic neuroma. Paper read at V symposium of International ERA study group. Jerusalem.

Gibson, W. P. R., Moffat, D. A. & Ramsden, R. T. (1977a) Clinical electrocochleography in the diagnosis and management of Ménière's disorder. *Audiology.* 16. 389-401.

Gibson, W. P. R., Ramsden, R. T. & Moffat, D. A. (1977b) The immediate effects of naftidrofuryl on the human electrocochleogram in Ménière's disorder—preliminary findings. *Journal of Laryngology and Otology.* 91. 679-696.

Gibson, W. P. R. & Wallace D. (1975) Basilar artery ectasia (an unusual cause of a cerebello-pontine angle lesion and hemifacial spasm. *Journal of Laryngology and Otology,* 89, 721-731.

Goff, W. R., Matsumiya, Y., Allison, T. & Goff, G. D. (1969) Cross-modality comparisons of averaged evoked potentials. In *Average Evoked Potentials: Methods, Results and Evaluations,* edited by E. Donchin, and D. Lindsley, pp. 95-141. *NASA SP 191.* Washington DC: US government printing office.

Goldstein, R. (1954) Analysis of summating potential in cochlear responses of guinea pigs. *American Journal of Physiology,* 178, 331-337.

Goldstein, R. (1965) Early components of the AER. *Acta Otolaryngologica,* supplementum 206, 127-128.

Goldstein, R. & Rodman, L. B. (1967) Early components of averaged evoked responses to rapidly repeated auditory stimuli. *Journal of Speech and Hearing Research,* 10, 697-705.

Graham, J. M,, Hutton, J. N. T. & Beagley, H. A. (1975) Post-auricular myogenic response during trans-tympanic electrocochleography (ECochG). *British Journal of Audiology,* 9, 116.

Greisen, O. & Rasmussen, P. E. (1970) Stapedius muscle reflexes and otoneurological examination in brain-stem tumours. *Acta Otolaryngologica,* 70, 366-370.

Hall, J. L. II. (1964) Binaural interaction in the accessory superior olivary nucleus of the cat. Technical report, no. 416. Research laboratory of electronics. Massachusetts Institute of Technology. Cambridge, Massachusetts: MIT press.

Halliday, A. M., McDonald, W. I. & Mushin, J. (1972) Delayed visual evoked response in eptic neuritis. *Lancet,* i, 982-985.

Hallpike, G. S. and Cairns, H. (1938) Observations on the pathology of Meniere's syndrome. *Journal of Laryngology and Otology,* 53, 625-655.

Harker, L. A., Hosick, E. C., Voots, R. J. & Mendel, M. I. (1977) Influence of succinylcholine on middle component auditory evoked potentials. *Archives of Otolaryngology,* 103, 133-137.

Harrison, J. M. & Irving, R. (1966) The organisation of the posterior ventral cochlear nucleus in rat. *Journal of Comparative Neurology,* **126,** 391-397.

Harrison, M. S. & Naftalin, L. (1968) *Menière's disease. Mechanism and Management.* Springfield: Charles C. Thomas.

Hazell, J. W. P., Conway, M., Fraser, J. G. & Keene, M. (1977) Audiological screening using the postaurical myogenic response and a machine scoring system. Paper read at V symposium of international ERA study group. Jerusalem.

Hecox, K. (1975) Electrophysiological correlates of human auditory development. In *Infant Perception,* edited by M. H. Cohen, and Salapatek. New York: Academic Press.

Hecox, K. & Galambos, R. (1974) Brainstem auditory evoked responses in human infants and adults. *Archives of Otolaryngology,* **99,** 30-33.

Helmholtz, H. L. F. (1859) Ueber physikalische ursurche der harmonie und disharmonie. *Gesellsch. deutsch Naturf Aertz,* **34,** 157-159.

Helmholtz, H. L. F. (1863) Die lehre von den to nempfindungen als physiologische grundlage für die theorie der musik. English translation in *On the Sensations of Tone,* edited by A. E. Ellis, (1875) London: Longmans & Green.

Hillyard, S. A. (1974) Methodological issues in CNV research. In *Bioelectric recording techniques, Part B, Electroencephalography and Human Brain Potentials,* edited by Thompson, R. F. & Patterson, M. Chapter 8. New York: Academic Press.

Hillyard, S. A. & Galambos, R. (1970) Eye-movement artefact in CNV. *Electroencephalography and Clinical Neurophysiology,* **28,** 173-182.

Hillyard, S. A., Hink, R. F., Schwent, V. L. & Picton, T. W. (1973) Electrical signs of selective attention in the human brain. *Science,* **182,** 177-180.

Hillyard, S. A., Squires, K. C., Bauer, J. W. & Lindsay, P. H. (1971) Evoked potential correlates of auditory signal detection. *Science,* **172,** 1357-1360.

Hood, D. C. (1974) Evoked cortical response audiometry. In *Physiological Measures of the Audio-vestibular System,* edited by L. J. Bradford, Chapter 10. New York: Academic Press.

Hoke, M. (1976) Problems of cochlear microphonic recording in man. *Revue de Laryngologie,* **97,** supplementum, 473-486.

Horowitz, S. F., Larson, S. J. & Sances, A. Jr. (1966) Evoked potentials as an adjunct to auditory evaluation of patients. In *Proceedings of the Symposium on Biomedical Engineering. I,* pp. 49-52. Milwaukee: Marquette University.

Humphries, K. N., Ashcroft, P. B. & Douek, E. E. (1977) Extra-tympanic electrocochleography. *Acta Otolaryngologica,* **83,** 303-309.

Humphries, K. N., Gibson, W. P. R. & Douek, E. E. (1976) Objective methods of hearing assessment: a system for recording the crossed acoustic response. *Medical and Biological Engineering,* **42,** 1-7.

Hutton, J. N. T. (1976) Anaesthesia for electrocochleography. *Clinical Otolaryngology,* **1,** 39-44.

Hyde, M. L. (1976) Properties of the auditory evoked vertex response in man. Unpublished PHD thesis: University of London.

Ilberg, von. (1968) Elektronenmikroskopische. Untersuchungen über diffusion und resorption von thoriumdioxyd an der meerschweinchesnecke. 3limbus spiralis. *Archiv fur Klinische und Experimentelle Ohren—Nasen—und Kehlkopfheilkunde,* **192,** 163-175

Industrial injuries advisory council—report (1973) *Occupational Deafness.* London: H.M.S.O.

Irwin, D. A., Rebert, C. S., McAdam, D. W. & Knott, J. R. (1966) Slow potential changes (CNV) in the human EEG as a function of motivational variables. *Electroencephalography and Clinical Neurophysiology,* **21,** 412-413.

Iwata, H., Tanahashi, T., Niwa, H., Tanaka, H., Koide, F. & Hamaguchi, S. (1976) Electrocochleographic study on sudden deafness. Paper read at XIII International Congress of Audiology. Florence.

Jacobson, J. L., Cody, D. T. R., Lambert, E. H. & Bickford, R. G. (1964) Physiological properties of the post-auricular response (sonomotor) in man. *Physiologist,* **7,** 167.

Jarcho, L. W. (1949) Excitability of cortical afferent systems during barbiturate anaesthesia. *Journal of Neurophysiology,* **12,** 447-457.

Jasper, H. H. (1958) The ten-twenty electrode system of the international federation. *Electroencephalography and Clinical Neurophysiology,* **10,** 371-375.

Jerger, S., Neely, J. G. & Jerger, J. (1975) Recovery of crossed acoustic reflexes in brain stem auditory disorder. *Archives of Otolaryngology,* **101,** 329-332.

Jewett, D. L. (1970) Volume-conducted potentials in response to auditory stimuli as detected by averaging in the cat. *Electroencephalography and Clinical Neurophysiology,* **28,** 609-618.

Jewett, D. L. & Romano, M. N. (1972) Neonatal development of auditory system potentials averaged from the scalp of rat and cat. *Brain Research,* **36,** 101-115.

Jewett, D. L., Romano, M. N. & Williston, J. S. (1970) Human auditory evoked potentials: possible brainstem components detected on the scalp. *Science,* **167,** 1517-1518.

Jewett, D. L. & Williston, J. S. (1971) Auditory-evoked far fields averaged from the scalp of humans. *Brain,* **94,** 681-696.

Johannsen, H. S. (1971) Elimination of movement artefacts in evoked response audiometry in infants. *Journal of Auditory Research,* **11,** 351-356.

Johnstone, B. M. & Boyle, A. L. F. (1967) Basilar membrane vibrations examined with the Mössbauer technique. *Science,* **158,** 389-390.

Jones, B. N., Scott, S. C. C., Binnie, C. D. & Roberts, J. R. (1975) Clinical and evoked response audiometry in late infancy. *Developmental Medicine and Child Neurology,,* **17,** 726-731.

Jungert, S. (1958) Auditory pathways in the brain stem. *Acta Otolaryngologica,* supplementum **138.**

Kado, R. T. & Adey, W. R. (1968) Electrode problems in central nervous monitoring in performing subjects. *Annals of the New York Academy of Science,* **148,** 263-278.

Karnahl, T. & Benning, C. D. (1972) Effect of sedation upon evoked response audiometry: amplitude and latency vs. sound pressure level. *Archiv Für Klinische und Experimentelle Ohren—Nasen—und Kehldopfheilkunde,* **201,** 181-188.

Katsuki, Y., Sumi, T., Uchiyama, H. & Watanabe, T. (1958) Electric response of auditory neurons in cat to sound stimulation. *Journal of Neurophysiology,* **21,** 569-588.

Kawamura, S., Ichikawa, G., Miyazaki, M. & Suetsuga, Y. (1972) The threshold measurement in relation to the proceedure of ERA. Paper read at XI International Congress of Audiology, Budapest.

Khechinashvili, S. N. & Kevanishvili Z. S. (1974) Experiences in computer audiology (ECoG and ERA) *Audiology,* **13,** 391-402.

Keidel, W. D. (1971a) DC potentials in auditory evoked response in man. *Acta Oto-laryngologica,* **71,** 242-248.

Keidel, W. D. (1971b) The use of quick correlators in electrocochleography; both in oto-audiography (OAG) and in neuro-audiography (NAG). *Revue de Laryngologie,* supplementum, 709-720.

Keidel, W. D. & Spreng, M. (1965) Neurophysiological evidence for the Stevens Power function in man. *Journal of the Acoustical Society of America,* **38,** 191-195.

Kiang, N. Y-S. (1955) An electrophysiological study of cat auditory cortex. Doctoral dissertation no. 3028. University of Chicago.

Kiang, N. Y-S. (1968) A survey of recent developments in the study of auditory physiology. *Annals of Otology, Rhinology and Laryngology,* **77,** 656-675.

Kiang, N. Y-S., Crist, A. H., French, M. A. & Edwards, A. G. (1963) Post-auricular electrical response to acoustic stimuli in humans. Quarterly progress report, no. 68. Research laboratory of electronics. Massachusetts Institute of Technology. Camrbidge, Massachusetts: MIT press.

Kiang, N. Y-S., Moxon, E. C. & Levine, R. A. (1970) Auditory-nerve activity in cats with normal and abnormal cochleas. In *CIBA Symposium on Sensorineural Hearing Loss* edited by G. E. W. Wolstenholme, and J. Knight, pp. 241-273. London: Churchill.

Kiang, N. Y-S. & Peake, W. T. (1960) Components of electrical responses recorded from the cochlea. *Annals of Otology, Rhinology and Laryngology,* **69,** 448-458.

Kiang, N. Y-S., Pfeiffer, R. R., Warr, W. B. & Backus, A. S. N. (1965) Stimulus coding in the cochlear nucleus. *Annals of Otology, Rhinology and Laryngology,* **74,** 463-485.

Kiang, N. Y-S., Watanabe, T., Thomas, E. C. & Clarke, L. F. (1965) Discharge patterns of single fibres in the cats auditory nerve. Research monograph, no. 35. Research laboratory of electronics. Massachusetts Institute of Technology. Cambridge, Massachusetts: MIT press.

King, T. T., Gibson, W. P. R. & Morrison, A. W. (1976) Tumours of the eighth cranial nerve. *British Journal of Hospital Medicine,* **16,** 259-272.

Knight, J. J. & Beagley, H. A. (1968) Auditory response and loudness function. *International Audiology,* **8,** 382-386.

Knott, J. R. & Irwin, D. A. (1968) Anxiety, stress and contingent negative variation. *Electroencephalography and Clinical Neurophysiology,* **24,** 286-287.

Knox, A. W. (1972) Electrodermal audiometry. In *Handbook of Clinical Audiology,* edited by J. Katz, pp. 395-406. Baltimore: Williams and Wilkins.

Köhler, W., Held, R. & O'Connell, D. N. (1952) An investigation of cortical currents. *Proceedings of the American Philosophical Society,* **96,** 290-330.

Köhler, W., & O'Connell, D. N. (1957) Currents of the visual cortex in the cat. *Journal of Cellular and Comparative Physiology,* **49,** supplement **2,** 1-43.

Kohllöffel, L. U. E. (1972) A study of basilar membrane vibrations III The basilar membrane frequency response curve in the living guinea pig. *Acustica,* **27,** 82-89.

Kooi, K. A., Tipton, A. C. & Marshall, R. E. (1971) Polarities and field configurations of the vertex components of the human evoked response: a reinterpretation. *Electroencephalography and Clinical Neurophysiology,* **31,** 166-169.

Kornhuber, H. H. & Deecke, L. (1965) Hirnpotentialänderungen bei willkürbewegungen und passiven bewegungen des menschen: bereitschaftspotential und reafferente potentiale. *Pfluegers Archiv für die Gesamte Physiologie des Mensch und der Tiere,* **284,** 1-17.

Kupperman, R. (1966) The dynamic dc potential in the cochlea of guinea pig (summating potential). *Acta Oto-laryngologica,* **62,** 465-480.

Kupperman, G. (1970) *Effects of three stimulus parameters on the early components of the averaged electroencephalic response.* Dissertation. University of Wisconsin.

Kupperman, G. L. & Mendel, M. I. (1974) Threshold of the early averaged electroencephalic response determined with tone pips and clicks during drug-induced sleep. *Audiology,* **13,** 379-390.

Lane, R. H., Kupperman, G. L. & Goldstein, R. (1971) Early components of the AER in relation to rise-decay time and duration of pure tones. *Journal of Speech and Hearing Research,* **14,** 408-415.

Lane, R. H., Mendel, M. I. & Kupperman, G. L. (1974) Phase distortion of the auditory AER imposed by analog filtering. *Archives of Otolaryngology,* **99,** 428-432.

Lawrence, M., Nuttal, A. L. and Clapper, M. P. (1974) Electrical potentials and fluid boundaries within the organ of Corti. *Journal of the Acoustical Society of America,* **55,** 122-138.

Lawrence, M. & McCabe, B. F. (1959) Inner ear mechanics and deafness; special considerations of Ménière's syndrome. *Journal of the American Medical Association,* **171,** 1927-1932

Leibman, J. & Graham, J. T. (1967) Changes in parameters of averaged auditory evoked potentials related to the number of data samples analyzed. *Journal of Speech and Hearing Research,* **10,** 782-785.

Lempert, J., Wever, E. G. & Lawrence, M. (1947) The cochleogram and its application. *Archives of Otolaryngology,* **45,** 61-67.

Lempert, J., Meltzer, P. E., Wever, E. G. & Lawrence, M. (1950) The cochleogram and its clinical application. *Archives of Otolaryngology,* **51,** 307-311.

Lev, A. & Sohmer, H. (1972) Sources of averaged neural responses recorded in animal and human subjects during cochlear audiometry (Electro-cochleogram). *Archiv fur Klinische und Experimentelle Ohren—Nasen—und Kehlkopfheilkunde,* **201,** 79-90.

Lewry, F. H. & Kobrak, H. (1936) The neural projection of the cochlear spirals on the primary acoustic centres. *Archives of Neurology and Psychiatry,* **35,** 839-852.

Lindsley, D. B. (1951) Emotion. In *Handbook of Experimental Psychology,* edited by S. S. Stevens, Chapter 14, pp. 473-516. New York: John Wiley.

Loomis, A. L., Harvey, E. N. & Hobart, G. (1938) Disturbance-patterns in sleep. *Journal of Neurophysiology,* **1,** 413-430.

Lorente de Nó, R. (1933a) Anatomy of the eighth nerve. I. The central projection of the nerve endings of the internal ear. *Laryngoscope,* **43,** 1-38.

Lorente de Nó, R. (1933b) Anatomy of the eighth nerve. III. General plan of structure of the primary cochlear nuclei. *Laryngoscope,* **43,** 327-350.

Low, M. D., Borda, R. P., Frost, J. D. Jr. & Kellaway, P. (1966a) Surface-negative, slow potential shift associated with conditioning in man. *Neurology,* **16,** 771-782.

Low, M. D., Frost, J. D., Borda, R. P. & Kellaway, P. (1966b) Surface negative slow potential shift associated with conditioning in man and sub-human primates. *Electroencephalography and Clinical Neurophysiology,* **21,** 413.

Lowell, E. L. (1965) In discussion of Davis, H. Sonomotor reflexes; myogenic evoked potentials. In *The Young Deaf Child: Identification and Management,* edited by H. Davis. *Acta Otolaryngologica,* supplementum **206,** 124-127.

Lowell, E. L., William, C. T., Ballinger, M. & Alvig, D. P. (1961) Measurement of auditory threshold with a special purpose analog computer. *Journal of Speech and Hearing Research,* **4,** 105-112.

Madell, J. R. & Goldstein, R. (1972) Relation between loudness and the amplitude of the early components of the averaged electroencephalic response. *Journal of Speech and Hearing Research,* **15,** 134-141.

Martin, J. L. & Coats, A. C. (1973) Short-latency auditory evoked responses, recorded from the human nasopharynx. *Brain Research,* **60,** 496-502.

Mast, T. E. (1963) Muscular vs cerebral sources for the short-latency human evoked responses to clicks. *Physiologist,* **6,** 229.

Mast, T. E. (1965) Short-latency human evoked responses to clicks. *Journal of Applied Physiology,* **20,** 725-730.

Mast, T. E. & Watson. C. (1968) Attention and auditory evoked responses to low detectability signals. *Perception and Psychophysics,* **4,** 237-240.

McAdam, D. W., Knott, J. R. & Rebert, C. S. (1969) Cortical slow potential changes in man related to interstimulus interval and to pre-trial prediction of interstimulus interval. *Psychophysiology,* **5,** 349-358.

McAdam, D. W. & Searle, D. M. (1969) Bereitschaftspotential enhancement with increased level of motivation. *Electroencephalography and Clinical Neurophysiology,* **27,** 73-75.

McCandless, G. A. (1967) Clinical application of evoked response audiometry. *Journal of Speech and Hearing Research,* **10,** 468-478.

McCandless, G. A. and Best, L. (1964) Evoked responses to auditory stimuli in men using a summing computer *Journal of Speech and Hearing Research,* **9,** 266-272.

McCandless, G. A. & Best, L. (1966) Summed evoked responses using pure tone stimuli. *Journal of Speech and Hearing. Research,* **9,** 266-272.

McCallum, W. C. & Walter, W. G. (1968) The effects of attention and distraction on the contingent negative variation in normal and neurotic subjects. *Electroencephalography and Clinical Neurophysiology,* **25,** 319-329.

Meir-Ewert, K., Gleitsmann, K. & Reiter, F. (1974) Acoustic jaw reflex in man; its relationship to other brain-stem and microreflexes. *Electroencephalography and Clinical Neurophysiology,* **36,** 629-637.

Mendel, M. I. (1975) Personal communication to Hood, D. C. Reported in evoked cortical response audiometry. In *Physiological Measures of the Audio-visual System,* edited by L. G. Bradford, Chapter 10. New York: Academic Press.

Mendel, M. I. (1974a) Influence of stimulus level and sleep stage on the early components of the averaged electroencephalic response to clicks during all-night sleep. *Journal of Speech and Hearing Research,* **17,** 5-17.

Mendel, M. I. (1974b) Personal communication.

Mendel, M. I., Adkinson, C. D. & Harker, L. A. (1975) Middle components of the auditory evoked potentials in infants. Paper read at IV symposium of International ERA Study Group, London.

Mendel, M. I. & Goldstein, R. (1969) Stability of the early components of the averaged electroencephalic response. *Journal of Speech and Hearing Research,* **12,** 351-361.

Mendel, M. I. & Goldstein, R. (1971) Early components of the averaged electroencephalic response to constant clicks during all-night sleep. *Journal of Speech and Hearing Research,* **14,** 829-840.

Mendel, M. I. & Hosick, E. C. (1975) Effects of secobarbital on the early components of the auditory evoked potentials. *Revue de Laryngologie,* **96,** 178-184.

Ménière, P. (1861) Memoire sur des lésions de l'orielle interne domnant lieu à des symptômes de congestion cérébrale apoplectiform. *Gazette Medicale de Paris,* **16,** 597-601.

Michelson, R. P. & Vincent, W. R. (1975) Auditory evoked frequency following response in man. *Archives of Otolaryngology,* **101,** 6-10.

Milner, B. A. (1970) *The physical study of bioelectric potentials generated in response to acoustic stimuli.* Unpublished PHD Thesis. London University.

Moffat, D. A. (1977) Transtympanic electrochleography during glycerol dehydration. Paper read at V symposium of International ERA study group, Jerusalem.

Mokotoff, B., Schulman-Galambos, C. & Galambos, R. (1977) Brainstem auditory evoked responses in children. *Archives of Otolaryngology,* **103,** 28-42.

Moore, E. J. (1972) Peripheral electrophysiological responses in man to auditory stimuli. *Central Wisconsin Colony and Training School Research Proceedings,* **9.** supplementum 2.

Montandon, P. B., Megill, N. D., Kahn, A. R., Peake, W. T. & Kiang, N. Y-S. (1975a) Recording auditory-nerve potentials as an office proceedure. *Annals of Otology, Rhinology and Laryngology,* **84,** 2-10.

Montandon, P. B., Shepard, N. T., Marr, E. M., Peake, W. T. & Kiang, N. Y-S. (1975b) Auditory-nerve potentials from ear canals of patients with otologic problems. *Annals of Otology, Rhinology and Laryngology,* **84,** 164-174.

Morest, D. K. (1964) The neuronal architecture of the medial geniculate body of the cat. *Journal of Anatomy,* **98,** 611-630.

Morrell, F. (1965) Clinical neurology: some applications of scanning by computer. *Californian Medical Journal,* **103,** 406-416.

Morrison, A. W. (1976) The surgery of vertigo: saccus drainage for idiopathic endolymphatic hydrops. *Journal of Laryngology and Otology,* **90,** 87-93.

Morrison, A. W. & Booth, J. B. (1970) Sudden deafness: an otological emergency. *British Journal of Hospital Medicine,* **4,** 287-298.

Morrison, A. W., Gibson, W. P. R. & Beagley, H. A. (1976) Trans-tympanic electrocochleography in the diagnosis of retro-cochlear tumours. *Clinical Otolaryngology,* **1,** 153-167.

Moushegian, G., Rupert, A. L. & Stillman, R. D. (1973) Scalp recorded early responses in man to frequencies in the speech range. *Electroencephalography and Clinical Neurophysiology,* **35,** 665-667.

Moushegian, G., Rupert, A. L. & Whitcomb, M. A. (1964) Medial superior-olivary-unit response patterns to monaural and binaural clicks. *Journal of the Acoustical Society of America,* **36,** 196-202.

Munson, W. A. (1947) The growth of auditory sensation. *Journal of the Acoustical Society of America,* **19,** 584-589.

Naunton, R. F. & Zerlin, S. (1976) Human whole-nerve response to clicks of various frequencies. *Audiology,* **15,** 1-9.

Niemer, W. T. & Cheng, S. K. (1949) The ascending auditory system, a study of retrograde degeneration. *Anatomical Record,* **103,** 490.

Odenthal, D. W. & Eggermont, J. J. (1974) Clinical electrocochleography. In *Electrocochleography: Basic Principles and Clinical Application,* edited by J. J. Eggermont, D. W., Odenthal, P. H. Schmidt, and A. Spoor, *Acta Oto-laryngologica,* supplementum **316,** 62-74.

Odenthal, D. W. & Eggermont, J. J. (1976) Topodiagnostic value of electrocochleography in pontine angle tumours. Paper read at XIIIth International Congress of Audiology, Florence.

Odenthal, D. W., Eggermont, J. J. & Hermans, J. (1974) Diagnosis by electrocochleography. *Revue de Laryngologie,* **95,** 481-490.

Onishi, S. & Davis, H. (1968) Effects of duration and rise time of tone bursts on evoked potentials. *Journal of the Acoustical Society of America,* **44,** 582-591.

Osterhammel, P. A., Davis, H., Wier, C. C. & Hirsch, S. K. (1973) Adult auditory evoked vertex potential in sleep. *Audiology,* **12,** 116-128.

Osterhammel, P. A., Terkildsen, K. & Arndal, P. (1970) Evoked responses to SISI stimuli. Contralateral masking effects. *Acta Otolaryngologica,* supplementum **263,** 245-247.

Ozdamer, O. & Dallos, P. (1976) Input-output functions of cochlear whole-nerve action potentials: interpretation in terms of one population of neurones. *Journal of the Acoustical Society of America,* **59,** 143-147.

Papez, J. W. (1930) Superior olivary nucleus: its fibre connections. *Archives of Neurology and Psychiatry,* **24,** 1-20.

Parker, D. J. (1976) Derived 'high pass' brainstem responses. Paper read at 2nd meeting of British ERA Study Group, London.

Pavlov, I. P. (1927) *Conditioned Reflexes,* (translated by G. V. Anrep,) London: Oxford University Press.

Perlman, H. B. & Case, T. J. (1941) Electrical phenomena of the cochlea in man. *Archives of Otolaryngology,* **34,** 710-718.

Peters, J. F. & Mendel, M. I. (1974) Early components of the averaged electroencephalic response to monaural and binaural stimulation. *Audiology,* **13,** 195-204.

Picton, T. W. & Hillyard, S. A. (1972) Cephalic skin potentials in electroencephalography. *Electroencephalography and Clinical Neurophysiology,* **33,** 419-424.

Picton, T. W. & Hillyard, S. A. (1974) Human auditory evoked potentials II: Effects of attention. *Electroencephaolography and Clinical Neurophysiology,* **36,** 191-199.

Picton, T. W., Hillyard, S. A., Krausz, H. I. & Galambos, R. (1974) Human auditory evoked potentials I: Evaluation of components. *Electroencephalography and Clinical Neurophysiology,* **36,** 179-190.

Pignatro, O. (1972) Early evoked potentials by sound stimuli. Paper read at XI International Congress of Audiology. Budapest.

Portmann, M. (1977) Clinical electrocochleography. *Journal of Laryngology and Otology.* In press.

Portmann, M., Aran, J-M. & LeBert, G. (1968) Electro-cochléogramme humain en dehors de toute intervention chirurgicale. *Acta Oto-laryngologica,* **71,** 253-261.

Portmann, M., LeBert, G. & Aran, J-M. (1967) Potentiels cochleares obtenus chez l'homme en dehors de toute intervention chirurgicale. *Revue de Laryngologie*, **88**, 157-164.

Pratt, H. & Sohmer, H. (1975) Rate and intensity functions of cochlear and brainstem evoked response to click stimuli. Paper read at IVth Symposium of the International ERA Study Group. London.

Prevec, T. S., Lokar, J. & Cernelc, S. (1974) The use of CNV audiometry. *Audiology*, **13**, 447-457.

Pevec, T. S., Ribaric, K. & Butinar, D. (1977) The possibilities of the CNV-audiometry in children. Paper read at V symposium of the International ERA study group, Jerusalem.

Preyer, W. (1881) *Die Seele des Kindes* Leipzig: T. Grieber (English translation (1888) New York: Appleton and Co.).

Price, L. L., Rosenblut, B., Goldstein, R. & Shepherd D. C. (1966) The averaged evoked response to auditory stimulation. *Journal of Speech and Hearing Research*, **9**, 361-370.

Purser, D. & Whitfield, I. C. (1972) W-shaped excitatory-inhibitory response curves from the medial geniculate nucleus of the unanaesthetised cat. *Journal of Physiology*, **221**, 17P-18P.

Ramsden, R. T. (1977) personal communication.

Ramsden, R. T., Gibson, W. P. R. & Moffat, D. A. (1977) Anaesthesia of the tympanic membrane using iontophoresis. *Journal of Laryngology and Otology*. **91**, 779-785.

Ramsden, R. T., Moffat, D. A. & Gibson, W. P. R. (1977) Trans-tympanic electrocochleography in patients with syphilis and hearing loss. *Annals of Otology, Rhinology and Laryngology*. In press.

Ramsden, R. T., Wilson, P. & Gibson, W. P. R. (1977) Immediate electrocochleographic changes following intravenous infusion of Tobramycin. *Annals of Otology, Rhinology and Laryngology*. In press.

Rapin, I. & Bergman, M. (1969) Auditory evoked responses in uncertain diagnoses. *Archives of Otolaryngology*, **90**, 307-314.

Rapin, I. & Graziani, L. J. (1967) Auditory evoked responses in normal, brain-damaged and deaf infants. *Neurology*, **17**, 881-894.

Rapin, I., Schimmel, H., Tourk, L. M., Krasnegor, N. A. & Pollack, C. (1966) Evoked responses to clicks and tones of varying intensity in waking adults. *Electroencephalography and Clinical Neurophysiology*, **21**, 335-344.

Rapin, I., Tourk, L. M., Krasnegor, N. A. & Schimmel, H. (1965) A parametric study of auditory evoked response in normal waking adults—a preliminary report. *Acta Oto-laryngologica*. supplementum **206**, 113-117.

Rasmussen, G. L. (1942) An efferent cochlear bundle. *Anatomical Records*, **82**, 441.

Rasmussen, G. L. (1946) Olivary peduncle and other fibre projections of the superior olivary complex. *Journal of Comparative Neurology*, **84**, 141-219.

Rasmussen, G. L. (1960) Efferent fibres of the cochlear nerve and cochlear nucleus. In *Neural Mechanisms of the Auditory and Vestibular Systems*, edited by G. L. Rasmussen, and W. F. Windle, Springfield: Thomas.

Rebert, C. S. & Knott, J. R. (1970) The vertex nonspecific evoked potential and latency of contingent negative variation. *Electroencephalography and Clinical Neurophysiology*, **28**, 561-565.

Reneau, J. P. & Hnatiow, G. Z. (1975) *Evoked Response Audiometry: a Topical and Historical Review*. Baltimore: University Press.

Reneau, J. P. & Mast, R. (1968) Telemetric EEG audiometry instrumentation for use with the profoundly retarded. *American Journal of Mental Deficiency*, **72**, 506-511.

Report by the Industrial Injuries Advisory Council (1973) *Occupational Deafness*. London: HMSO.

Rioch, D. McK. (1929) Studies on the diencephalon of carnivora. I. The nuclear configuration of the thalamus, epithalamus and hypothalamus of the dog and cat. *Journal of Comparative Neurology*, **49**, 1-119.

Ritvo, E. R., Ornitz, E. M. & Walter, R. D. (1967) Clinical application of auditory averaged evoked response at sleep onset in the diagnosis of deafness. *Paedatrics*, **40**, 1003-1008.

Robinson, K. & Rudge, P. (1975) Auditory evoked responses in multiple sclerosis. *The Lancet*, **i**, 1164-1166.

Robinson, K. & Rudge, P. (1977) Abnormalities of the auditory system in patients with multiple sclerosis. *Brain*, **100**, 19-40.

Roeser, R. J., Price, L. L. and Hnatiow, G. Z. (1971) Evoked response audiometry, psychiatric patients. *Archives of Otolaryngology*, **94**, 208-213.

Ronis, B. J. (1966) Cochlear potentials in otosclerosis. *Laryngoscope*, **76**, 212-231.

Rose, D. E., Keating, L. W., Hedgecock, L. D., Miller, K. E. & Schreurs, K. K. (1972) A comparison of evoked response audiometry and routine clinical audiometry. *Audiology,* **11,** 238-243.

Rose, D. E. & Rittmanic, P. A. (1968) Evoked response tests with mentally retarded. *Archives of Otolaryngology,* **88,** 495-498.

Rose, D. E. & Ruhm, H. B. (1966) Some characteristics of the peak latency and amplitude of the acoustically evoked response. *Journal of Speech and Hearing Research,* **9,** 412-422.

Rose, J. E. (1949) The cellular structure of the auditory region of the cat. *Journal of Comparative Neurology,* **91,** 409-439.

Rose, J. E., Galambos, R. & Hughes, J. R. (1959) Microelectrode studies of the cochlear nuclei of the cat. *Bulletin of the John Hopkins Hospital,* **104,** 211-251.

Rose, J. E., Greenwood, D. D., Goldberg, J. M. & Hind, J. E. (1963) Some discharge characteristics of single neurones in the inferior colliculus of the cat. I. Tonotopical organisation, relation of spike-counts to tone intensity, and firing patterns of single elements. *Journal of Neurophysiology,* **26,** 294-320.

Rose, J. E. & Woolsey, C. N. (1949) The relations of thalamic connections, cellular structure and evokable electrical activity in the auditory region of the cat. *Journal of Comparative Neurology,* **91,** 441-446.

Rothman, H. H. (1970) Effects of high frequencies and intersubject variability on the auditory evoked cortical response. *Journal of the Acoustical Society of America,* **47,** 569-573.

Rousseau, J. C., Bostem, F. & Dongier, M. (1968) Studies on CNV: interest of recording its progressive construction during summation. *Electroencephalography and Clinical Neurophysiology,* **24,** 95.

Rowland, V. (1961) Electrographic responses in sleeping conditioned animals. In *The Nature of Sleep,* edited by G. E. W. Wolstenholm, and C. M. O'Conner. pp. 284-304. Boston: Littlebrown.

Rowland, V. & Goldstone, M. (1963) Appetively conditioned and drive-related bioelectric baseline shift in cat cortex. *Electroencephalography and Clinical Neurophysiology,* **15,** 474-485.

Rubel, E. W. & Parks, T. N. (1975) Organization and development of brain stem auditory nuclei of the chicken: Tonotopic organization of N. magnocellaris and N. laminaris. *Journal of Comparative Neurology,* **164,** 411-434.

Ruben, R. J., Bordley, J. E. & Lieberman, A. T. (1961) Cochlear potentials in man. *Laryngoscope,* **71,** 1141-1164.

Ruben, R. J., Sekula, J., Bordley, J. E., Knickerbocker, G. G., Nager, G. T. & Fisch, U. (1960) Human cochlear responses to sound stimuli. *Annals of Otology, Rhinology and Laryngology,* **69,** 459-476.

Ruben, R. J. & Walker, A. E. (1963) The VIIIth nerve action potential in Ménière's disease. *Laryngoscope,* **11,** 1456-1464.

Ruhm, H. & Flanigin, H. (1967) Acoustically-evoked potentials in man: mediation of early components. *Laryngoscope,* **77,** 806-822.

Rutherford, W. (1886) A new theory of hearing. *Journal of Anatomy and Physiology,* **21,** 166-168.

Salamy, A. & McKean, C. M. (1976) Postnatal development of human brainstem potentials during the first year of life. *Electroencephalography and Clinical Neurophysiology,* **40,** 418-426.

Salomon, G. (1975) A computer model for on-going EEG based on statistical data: clinical implications. Paper read at IVth Symposium of the International ERA Study Group, London.

Salomon, G. (1976) Personal communication.

Salomon, G., Beck, O. & Elberling, C. (1973) The role of sedation in ERA from the vertex. *Audiology,* **12,** 150-166.

Sando, I. (1965) The anatomical interrelationships of the cochlear nerve fibres. *Acta Oto-laryngologica,* **59,** 417-436.

Satterfield, J. H. (1966) A system for selection of responses for averaging. *Electroencephalography and Clinical Neurophysiology,* **21,** 86-88.

Saul, L. J. & Davis, H. A. (1932) Action currents in the central nervous system I. Action currents of the auditory tracts. *Archives of Neurology and Psychiatry,* **28,** 1104-1116.

Sayers, B. McA., Beagley, H. A. & Henshall, W. R. (1974) The mechanism of auditory evoked EEG responses. *Nature,* **247,** 481-483.

Schmidt, P. H., Eggermont, J. J. & Odenthal, D. W. (1974) Study of Ménière's disease by electrocochleography. *Acta Oto-laryngologica,* supplementum **316,** 75-84.

Schmidt, P. H., Odenthal, D. W., Eggermont, J. J. & Spoor, A. (1975) Electrocochleographic study of a case of Lermoyez's syndrome. *Acta Oto-laryngologica,* **79,** 287-291.

Schulman-Galambos, C. & Galambos, R. (1975) Brain stem auditory evoked responses in premature infants. *Journal of Speech and Hearing Research* **18,** 456-465.

Sem-Jacobsen, C. W., Petersen, M. C., Dodge, H. W. Jr., Lazarte, J. A. & Holman, C. B. (1956)

Electroencephalographic rhythms from the depths of the parietal, occipital and temporal lobes in man. *Electroencephalography and Clinical Neurophysiology,* **8,** 263-278.

Setters, W. A. & Brackmann, D. (1977) Acoustic tumour detection with brainstem electric response audiometry. *Annals of Otology, Rhinology and Laryngology.* **103,** 181-187.

Sharrard, G. A. W. (1973) Further conclusions regarding the influence of word meaning on the cortical averaged evoked response in audiology. *Audiology,* **12,** 103-115.

Shepard, D. C., Wever, O. E. & McCarren, K. (1970) Techniques to reduce the negative effects of high voltage electrical artefacts during averaged electroencephalic audiometry (AEA). *Journal of Speech and Hearing Disorders,* **35,** 142-155.

Shimizu, H. (1968) Evoked response in VIIIth nerve lesions. *Laryngoscope,* **78,** 2140-2151.

Simmons, F. B. & Beatty, D. L. (1962) The significance of RW-recorded cochlear potentials in hearing. *Annals of Otology, Rhinology and Laryngology,* **71,** 767-780.

Skinner, P. H. (1972) Electroencephalic response audiometry. In *Handbook of Clinical Audiology,* edited by J. Katz, Ch. 22, pp. 407-433. Baltimore: Williams & Wilkins.

Skinner, P. H. & Antinoro, F. (1969) Auditory evoked response in normal hearing adults and children ebfore and during sedation. *Journal of Speech and Hearing Research,* **12,** 394-401.

Skinner, P. H. & Antinoro, F. (1971) The effects of signal rise time and duration of the early components of the auditory evoked cortical response. *Journal of Speech and Hearing Research,* **14,** 552-558.

Skinner, P. H., Antinoro, F. & Shimota, J. (1974) An evaluation of linear extrapolation to threshold in electroencephalic response audiometry. *Journal of Auditory Research,* **12,** 26-31.

Skinner, P. H. & Jones, H. C. (1968) Effects of signal duration and rise time on the auditory evoked potential. *Journal of Speech and Hearing Research,* **11,** 301-306.

Skinner, P. H. & Shimota, J. (1973) Binaural summation and the early components of the auditory electroencephalic response. *Journal of Auditory Research,* **12,** 32-35.

Smith, C. A. & Dempsey, E. W. (1957) Electron microscopy of the organ of Corti. *American Journal of Anatomy,* **100,** 337-

Smith, C. A. & Sjöstrand, F. S. (1961) Structure of the nerve endings on the external hair cells of the guinea pig as studied by serial sections. *Journal of Ultrastructure Research,* **5,** 523-556.

Snider, R. S. & Stowell, A. (1944) Receiving areas of the tactile, auditory and visual systems in the cerebellum. *Journal of Neurophysiology,* **7,** 331-357.

Sohmer, H. (1973) Personal communication.

Sohmer, H. & Feinmesser, M. (1964) Cochlear potentials from cat tympanic membrane. *Life Sciences,* **13,** 1191-1194.

Sohmer, H. & Feinmesser, M. (1967) Cochlear action potentials recorded from the external ear in man. *Annals of Otology, Rhinology and Laryngology,* **76,** 427-435.

Sohmer, H. & Feinmesser, M. (1970) Cochlear and cortical audiometry conveniently recorded in the same subject. *Israel Journal of Medical Sciences,* **6,** 219-223.

Sohmer, H. & Feinmesser, M. (1971) Recording of averaged cochlear action potentials as a form of objective audiometry. Paper read at VII International Congress on Acoustics. Budapest.

Sohmer, H. & Feinmesser, M. (1973) Routine use of electrocochleography (cochlear audiometry) on human subjects. *Audiology,* **12,** 167-173.

Sohmer, H., Feinmesser, M. & Szabo, G. (1974) Sources of electrocochleographic responses as studied in patients with brain damage. *Electroencephalography and Clinical Neurophysiology,* **37,** 663-669.

Sohmer, H. & Tell, L. (1975) Cochlear brain-stem and cortical responses in non-organic hearing loss (NOHL). Paper read at IVth Symposium of the International ERA Study Group, London.

Spillman, T., Erdmann, W. & Leitner, H. (1975) Clinical experiences with Althesin sedation for ERA. *Revue de Laryngologie,* **96,** 192-197.

Spoendlin, H. (1966) The organisation of the cochlear receptor. *Advances in Oto-Rhino-Laryngology,* **13,** 1-227.

Spoendlin, H. (1970) Structural basis of peripheral frequency analysis. In *Frequency Analysis and Periodicity Detection in Hearing,* edited by R. Plomp, and F. G. Smoorenburg. pp. 2-36. Leiden, Sijthoff.

Spoendlin, H. (1972) Innervation densities of the cochlea. *Acta Oto-laryngologica,* **73,** 235-248.

Spoendlin, H. (1976) Organisation of the Auditory Receptor. *Revue de Laryngologie,* **97,** supplementum, 453-462.

Spoor, A (1974) Apparatus for electrocochleography. *Acta Oto-laryngologica,* supplementum 316, 25-36.

Spreng, M. (1969) Problems in objective cerebral audiometry using short sound stimuli. *International Audiology,* **8,** 424-429.

Spreng, M. (1974) Objective electrophysiological measurements of ear-characteristics, intelligibility of vowels and judgement of the stage of attention. AGARD conference pre-print, **152**, A6/1-10.

Spreng, M. & Keidel, W. D. (1967) Separierung von cerebroaudiogram (CAG), neuroaudiogramm (NAG) und otoaudiogram (OAG) in der objecktiven audiometry. *Archiv fur Klinische und Experimentelle Ohren—Nasen—und Kehlkopfheilkunde*, **189**, 225-246.

Squires, K. C., Hillyard, S. A. & Lindsay, P. H. (1973) Vertex potentials during auditory signal detection: relation to decision criteria. *Perception and Psychophysics*, **2**, 265-272.

Stange, G. (1972) The effect of sedative agents in psychotropic drugs on the acoustically evoked responses. *Archiv fur Klinische und Experimentelle Ohren—Nasen—und Kehlkopfheilkunde*, **201**, 294-308.

Stange, G. Spreng M, Keidel, Die wirkung von streptmycinsulfat auf erregung und adaption der haarzellen des cortischen organs. *Pfluegers Archiv fur die Gesamte Physiologie des Menschen und der Tiere*, **279**, 99-120.

Starr, A. & Achor, L. J. (1975) Auditory brainstem responses in neurological disease. *Archives of Neurology*, **32**, 761-768.

Starr, A. & Achor, L.J. (1977) Mapping the generators of the brainstem potentials. Paper read at the fifth symposium of the International ERA study group, Jerusalem.

Starr, A. & Hamilton, A. E. (1976) Correlation between confirmed sites of neurological lesions and abnormalities of far-field auditory brainstem responses. *Electroencephalography and Clinical Neurophysiology*, **41**, 595-608.

Steinberg, D. & Lehnhart, E. (1972) Impedanzbefunde bei zentralen horstorungen. *Zeitschrift fur Laryngologie, Rhinologie Otologie und ihre Grezgebiete*, **51**, 693-699.

Stopp, P. E. (1967) An 'afterpotential' in the cochlear response. *Nature*, **215**, 1400.

Stopp, P. E. & Whitfield, I. C. (1961) Unit responses from brainstem nuclei in the pidgeon. *Journal of Physiology*, **158**, 165-177.

Stopp, P. E. & Whitfield, I. C. (1964) Summating potentials in the avian cochlear. *Journal of Physiology*, **175**, 45-46.

Stotler, W. A. (1953) An experimental study of the cells and connections of the superior olivary complex of the cat. *Journal of Comparative Neurology*, **98**, 401-431.

Suzuki, T. (1975) *Recording the Brainstem Evoked Response: A Manual (preliminary draft)*, edited by C. Schulman-Galambos, R. Galambos, and T. Suzuki. Copenhagen: Madsen Electronics Ltd.

Suzuki, T. & Taguchi, K. (1965) Cerebral evoked response to auditory stimuli in waking man. *Annals of Otology, Rhinology and Laryngology*, **74**, 128-139.

Suzuki, T., Tanaka, Y. & Arayama, T. (1966) Detection of hearing disorders in children under three years of age. *International Audiology*, **5**, 74-76.

Tabor, J. R., Best, La Var G. & Metz, M. J. (1968) Vestibular testing by evoked response. *Audiology*, **7**, 429-430.

Tarchanoff, I. V. (1890) Uber die galvanischen erscheinungen in der haut des menschen bei reizungen der sinnesorgane und bei verschiedenen formen der psychischen thätigkeit. *Archiv für die gesamte Physiologie ees Menschens und der Tiere*, **14**, 46-55.

Tasaki, I. (1954) Nerve impulses in individual auditory nerve fibres of guinea pig. *Journal of Neurophysiology*, **17**, 97-122.

Tasaki, I., Davis, H. & Eldredge, D. H. (1954) Exploration of cochlear potentials in guinea pig with a microelectrode. *Journal of the Acoustical Society of America*, **26**, 765-773.

Tasaki, I., Davis, H. & Legouix, J-P. (1952) The space-time pattern of the cochlear microphonics (guinea pig) as recorded by differential electrodes. *Journal of the Acoustical Society of America*, **24**, 502-519.

Tasaki, I. & Spyropoulos, C. S. (1959) Stria vascularis as a source of endocochlear potential. *Journal of Neurophysiology*, **22**, 149-155.

Teas, D. C., Davis, H. & Legouix, J-P. (1962) The space-time pattern of the cochlear microphonic (guinea pig) as recorded by differential electrodes. *Journal of the Acoustical Society of America*, **34**, 1438-1459.

Teas, D. C., Eldredge, D. H. & Davis, H. (1962) Cochlear responses to acoustic transients: an interpretation of the whole-nerve action potentials. *Journal of the Acoustical Society of America*, **34**, 1438-1459.

Teas, D. C. & Kiang, N. Y-S. (1964) Evoked responses from the auditory cortex. *Experimental Neurology*, **10**, 91-119.

Terkildsen, K. (1975) Personal communication.

Terkildsen, K., Osterhammel, P. & Huis In't Veld, F. (1973) Electrocochleography with a far field technique. *Scandanavian Audiology,* **2,** 141-148.

Terkildsen, K., Osterhammel, P. & Huis In't Veld, F. (1975) Far-field electrocochleography. Frequency specificity of the response. *Scandanavian Audiology,* **4,** 167-172.

Terkildsen, K., Osterhammel, P. & Huis In't Veld, F. (1976) Far-field electrocochleography. Adaptation. *Scandanavian Audiology,* **4,** 215-220.

Thornton, A.R.D. (1974) Statistical properties of electrocochleographic responses and their use in clinical diagnosis. Paper read at International Conference on Electrocochleography. Albert Einstein College of Medicine. New York.

Thornton, A. R. D. (1975a) The diagnostic potential of surface recorded electrocochleography. *British Journal of Audiology,* **9,** 7-13.

Thornton, A. R. D. (1975b) Bilaterally recorded early acoustic responses. *Scandanavian Audiology,* **4,** 173-181.

Thornton, A. R. D. (1975c) Distortion of averaged post-auricular muscle responses due to system bandwidth limits. *Electroencephalography and Clinical Neurophysiology,* **39,** 195-197.

Thornton, A. R. D. (1975d) The use of post-auricular muscle responses. *Journal of Laryngology and Otology,* **89,** 997-1010.

Thornton, A. R. D. (1976a) Electrophysiological studies of the auditory system. *Audiology,* **15,** 23-38.

Thornton, A. R. D. (1976b) Properties of auditory brainstem evoked responses. *Revue de Laryngologie,* **97,** supplementum, 591-602.

Thornton, A. R. D. & Coleman, M. J. (1975) The adaptation of cochlear and brainstem auditory evoked potentials. *Electroencephalography and Clinical Neurophysiology,* **39,** 399-406.

Thornton, A. R. D. & Hawkes, C. H. (1976a) Neurological applications of surface-recorded electrocochleography. *Journal of Neurology, Neurosurgery and Psychiatry,* **39,** 586-592.

Thornton, A. R. D. & Hawkes, C. H. (1976b) Cochlear and brainstem evoked responses in multiple sclerosis. Paper read at XIIIth International Congress of Audiology, Florence.

Tonndorf, J. (1962) Time/frequency analysis along the partition of cochlear-models. A modified concept. *Journal of the Acoustical Society of America,* **34,** 1337-1350.

Totsuka, G., Nakamura, K. & Kirikae, I. (1954) Studies of the acoustic reflex. Part I Electromyographic studies of the acousti-auricular reflex. *Annals of Otology, Rhinology and Laryngology,* **63,** 939-949.

Townsend, G. L. & Cody, D. T. R. (1970) Vertex response: influence of lesions in the auditory system. *Laryngoscope,* **80,** 979-999.

Townsend, G. L. & Cody, D. T. R. (1971) The averaged inion response evoked by acoustic stimulation: its relation to the saccule. *Annals of Otology, Rhinology and Laryngology,* **80,** 121-131.

Tyberghein, J. & Forrez, G. (1969) Cortical audiometry in normal hearing subjects. *Acta Otolaryngologica,* **67,** 24-32.

Utsumi, S., Inui, Y & Inui, O. (1966) An objective hearing test by means of auditory electro-oculomotography (AOG). *International Audiology,* **5,** 230-233.

Uziel, A. (1975) Electrophysiological study of auditory recruitment by ERA. Paper read at IVth Symposium of International ERA Study Group, London.

Vaughan, H. G. (1969) The relationship of brain activity to scalp recordings of event-related potentials. In *Averaged Evoked Potentials,* edited by E. Donchin, and D. B. Lindsley. NASA SP-191, chapter 2. Washington: US Government printing office.

Vaughan, H. G., Costa, L. D. & Ritter, W. (1968) Topography of the human motor potential. *Electroencephalography and Clinical Neurophysiology,* **25,** 1-10.

Vaughan, H. G. & Ritter, W. (1970) The sources of auditory evoked response recorded from the human scalp. *Electroencephalography and Clinical Neurophysiology,* **28,** 360-367.

Ventry, I. M. (1975) Conditioned galavanic skin response audiometry. In *Physiological Measures of the Audio-vestibular System,* edited by L. G. Bradford, Chapter 7. New York: Academic Press.

Vigouroux, R. (1879) Sur le rôle de la resistance électrique dans l'ectro-diagnostic. *Gazette Medicale,* **51,** 657-658. (Paris)

Walter, H. (1964a) The convergence and interaction of visual, auditory and tactile responses in human nonspecific cortex. *Annals of the New York Academy of Science,* **112,** 320-361.

Walter, W. G. (1964b) Slow potential waves in the human brain associated with expectancy, attention and decision. *Archives of Psychiatry,* **206,** 309-322.

Walter, W. G. (1966) Electrophysiologic contributions to psychiatric therapy. *Current Psychiatric Therapeutics*, **6**, 13-25.

Walter, W. G. (1967) Electrical signs of association, expectancy and decision in the human brain. *Electroencephalography and Clinical Neurophysiology, supplement* **25**, 258-263.

Walter, W. G., Aldridge, V. J., Cooper, R., McCallum, C. & Cohen, J. (1965) The interaction of responses to semantic stimuli in the human brain. *Electroencephalography and Clinical Neurophysiology*, **18**, 514-515.

Walter, W. G., Cooper, R., Aldridge, V. J., McCallum, W. C. & Winter, A. L. (1964) Contingent negative variation: an electric sign of sensorimotor association and expectancy in the human brain. *Nature*, **203**, 380-384.

Walter, W. G., Cooper, R., McCallum, C. & Cohen, J. (1965) The origin and significance of the contingent negative variation or "expectancy wave". *Electroencephalography and Clinical Neurophysiology*, **18**, 720.

Wang, C. W. (1954) Quoted by Miller, M. H. & Polisar, I. A. (1964) In *Audiological Evaluation of the Paedatric Patient* edited by R. West, Ch. 4, p. 52. Springfield: Charles C. Thomas.

Weitzman, E. D., Graziani, L. & Duhamel, L. (1967) Maturation and topography of the auditory evoked response of the prematurely born infant. *Electroencephalography and Clinical Neurophysiology*, **23**, 82-83.

Wever, E. G. (1949) *Theory of Hearing*. New York: John Wiley & Sons, Inc.

Wever, E. G. & Bray, C. W. (1930) Action currents in the auditory nerve in response to acoustic stimulation. *Proceedings of the National Academy of Science, U.S.A.*, **16**, 344-350.

Wever, E. G. & Lawrence, M. (1954) *Physiological Acoustics*. Princeton: Princeton University Press.

Wever, E. G. & Vernon, J. A. (1960) The problem of hearing in snakes. *Journal of Auditory Research*, **1**, 77-83.

Whitfield, I. C. (1956) Electrophysiology of the central auditory pathway. *British Medical Bulletin*, **12**, 105-109.

Whitfield, I. C. (1967) *The Auditory Pathway*. London: Edward Arnold.

Whitfield, I. C. & Ross, H. F. (1965) Cochlear-microphonic and summating potentials and the outputs of individual hair-cell generators. *Journal of the Acoustical Society of America*, **38**, 126-131.

Williams, W. G. & Graham, J. T. (1963) EEG responses to auditory stimuli in waking children. *Journal of Speech and Hearing Research*, **6**, 57-63.

Wilson, J. P. & Johnstone, J. R. (1975) Basilar membrane and middle ear vibration in guinea pig measured by capacitive probe. *Journal of the Acoustical Society of America*, **57**, 705-723.

Worden, F. G. & Marsh, J. T. (1968) Frequency-following (microphonic-like) neural responses evoked by sound. *Electroencephalography and Clinical Neurophysiology*, **25**, 42-52.

Wright, H. N. (1968) Clinical measurement of temporal auditory summation. *Journal of Speech and Hearing Research*, **11**, 109-127.

Wurtz, R. H. (1966) Steady potential correlates of intracranial reinforcement. *Electroencephalography and Clinical Neurophysiology*, **20**, 59-67.

Yamada, O., Yagi, T., Yamane, H. & Suzuki, J-I. (1975) Clinical evaluation of the auditory evoked brain stem response. *Auris. Nasus. Larynx*, **2**, 97-105.

Yoshie, N. (1968) Auditory nerve action potential responses to clicks in man. *Laryngoscope*, **178**, 198-215.

Yoshie, N. (1973) Diagnostic significance of the electrocochleogram in clinical audiometry. *Audiology*, **12**, 504-539.

Yoshie, N. & Okudaira, T. (1969) Myogenic evoked potential responses to clicks in man. *Acta Otolaryngologica*, supplementum 252, 89-103.

Yoshie, N., Ohashi, T. & Suzuki, T. (1967) Non-surgical recordings of auditory nerve action potentails in man. *Laryngoscope*, **77**, 76-85.

Yoshie, N. & Yamaura, K. (1969) Cochlear microphonic responses to pure tones in man recorded by a non-surgical method. *Acta Oto-laryngologica*. supplementum 252, 37-69.

Zerlin, S. (1969) Travelling wave velocity in the human cochlea. *Journal of the Acoustical Society of America*, **46**, 1011-1015.

Zerlin, S., Naunton, R. F. & Mowry, H. J. (1973) The early evoked cortical response to third-octave clicks and tones. *Audiology*, **12**, 242-249.

Zwicker, E. & Fast, L. (1972) On the developement of the critical band. *Journal of the Acoustical Soceity of America*, **52**, 699-702.

Zwislocki, J. J. (1960) Theory of temporal auditory summation. *Journal of the Acoustical Society of America,* **32,** 1046-1060.

Zwislocki, J. J. (1974) A possible neuro-mechanical sound analysis in the cochlea. *Acoustica,* **31,** 354-359.

Zwislocki, J. J. (1975) Phase opposition between inner and outer hair cells and auditory sound analysis, *Audiology,* **14,** 443-445.

Index

225